New Concepts in Diagnostic Imaging

Guest Editors

MARTHA MOON LARSON, DVM, MS
GREGORY B. DANIEL, DVM, MS

VETERINARY CLINICS OF NORTH AMERICA: SMALL ANIMAL PRACTICE

www.vetsmall.theclinics.com

July 2009 • Volume 39 • Number 4

SAUNDERS an imprint of ELSEVIER, Inc.

W.B. SAUNDERS COMPANY
A Division of Elsevier Inc.

1600 John F. Kennedy Blvd. ● Suite 1800 ● Philadelphia, PA 19103-2899

http://www.vetsmall.theclinics.com

**VETERINARY CLINICS OF NORTH AMERICA: SMALL ANIMAL PRACTICE Volume 39, Number 4
July 2009 ISSN 0195-5616, ISBN-13: 978-1-4377-1285-8, ISBN-10: 1-4377-1285-1**

Editor: John Vassallo; j.vassallo@elsevier.com
Developmental Editor: Theresa Collier

Veterinary Clinics of North America: Small Animal Practice (ISSN 0195-5616) is published bimonthly (For Post Office use only: volume 39 issue 4 of 6) by Elsevier Inc., 360 Park Avenue South, New York, NY 10010-1710. Months of issue are January, March, May, July, September, and November. Business and Editorial Offices: 1600 John F. Kennedy Blvd., Suite 1800, Philadelphia, PA 19103-2899. Customer Service Office: 11830 Westline Industrial Drive, St. Louis, MO 63146. Periodicals postage paid at New York, NY and additional mailing offices. Subscription prices are $229.00 per year (domestic individuals), $366.00 per year (domestic institutions), $114.00 per year (domestic students/residents), $303.00 per year (Canadian individuals), $450.00 per year (Canadian institutions), $336.00 per year (international individuals), $450.00 per year (international institutions), and $165.00 per year (international and Canadian students/residents). To receive student/resident rate, orders must be accompanied by name of affiliated institution, date of term, and the *signature* of program/residency coordinator on institution letterhead. Orders will be billed at individual rate until proof of status is received. Foreign air speed delivery is included in all *Clinics* subscription prices. All prices are subject to change without notice. **POSTMASTER:** Send address changes to *Veterinary Clinics of North America: Small Animal Practice*, 11830 Westline Industrial Drive, St. Louis, MO 63146. Customer Service (orders, claims, online, change of address): Elsevier Periodicals Customer Service, 11830 Westline Industrial Drive, St. Louis, MO 63146. Tel: 1-800-654-2452 (U.S. and Canada). Fax: 314-523-5170. E-mail: journalscustomerservice-usa@elsevier.com (for print support); journalsonlinesupport-usa@elsevier.com (for online support).

Reprints. For copies of 100 or more of articles in this publication, please contact the Commercial Reprints Department, Elsevier Inc., 360 Park Avenue South, New York, NY 10010-1710. Tel.: 212-633-3812; Fax: 212-462-1935; E-mail: reprints@elsevier.com.

Veterinary Clinics of North America: Small Animal Practice is also published in Japanese by Inter Zoo Publishing Co., Ltd., Aoyama Crystal-Bldg 5F, 3-5-12 Kitaaoyama, Minato-ku, Tokyo 107-0061, Japan.

Veterinary Clinics of North America: Small Animal Practice is covered in *Current Contents/Agriculture, Biology and Environmental Sciences, Science Citation Index, ASCA, MEDLINE/PubMed (Index Medicus), Excerpta Medica,* and *BIOSIS.*

Printed in the United States of America.

Contributors

GUEST EDITORS

MARTHA MOON LARSON, DVM, MS
Diplomate, American College of Veterinary Radiology; Professor of Radiology, Department of Small Animal Clinical Sciences, Virgina-Maryland Regional College of Veterinary Medicine, Virginia Tech University, Blacksburg, Virginia

GREGORY B. DANIEL, DVM, MS
Diplomate, American College of Veterinary Radiology; Professor, Department of Small Animal Clinical Sciences, Virginia-Maryland Regional College of Veterinary Medicine, Virginia Tech University, Blacksburg, Virginia

AUTHORS

LAURA J. ARMBRUST, DVM
Diplomate, American College of Veterinary Radiology; Associate Professor of Radiology, Department of Clinical Sciences, Kansas State University, College of Veterinary Medicine, Veterinary Medical Teaching Hospital, Manhattan, Kansas

DAVID S. BILLER, DVM
Diplomate, American College of Veterinary Radiology; Professor of Diagnostic Imaging, Department of Clinical Sciences, Kansas State University, College of Veterinary Medicine, Veterinary Medical Teaching Hospital, Manhattan, Kansas

ERIN L. BRINKMAN-FERGUSON, DVM
Diplomate, American College of Veterinary Radiology; Assistant Professor of Diagnostic Imaging, Department of Clinical Sciences, College of Veterinary Medicine, Mississippi State University, Mississippi State, Mississippi

GREGORY B. DANIEL, DVM, MS
Diplomate, American College of Veterinary Radiology; Professor and Head, Department of Small Animal Clinical Sciences, Virginia-Maryland Regional College of Veterinary Medicine, Virginia Tech University, Blacksburg, Virginia

DAVID A. JIMÉNEZ, DVM
Department of Clinical Sciences, Kansas State University, College of Veterinary Medicine, Veterinary Teaching Hospital, Manhattan, Kansas

MARTHA MOON LARSON, DVM, MS
Diplomate, American College of Veterinary Radiology; Professor of Radiology, Department of Small Animal Clinical Sciences, Virgina-Maryland Regional College of Veterinary Medicine, Virginia Tech University, Blacksburg, Virginia

PETER V. SCRIVANI, DVM
Diplomate, American College of Veterinary Radiology; Assistant Professor, Department of Clinical Sciences, Veterinary Medical Center, College of Veterinary Medicine, Cornell University, Ithaca, New York

ALLISON ZWINGENBERGER, DVM, MAS
Diplomate, American College of Veterinary Radiology; Diplomate, European College of Veterinary Diagnostic Imaging; Department of Surgical and Radiological Sciences, School of Veterinary Medicine, University of California, Davis, Davis, California

Contents

ensure appropriate security. A hospital information system or radiology information system can be used to tie the patient record with the digital images in a paperless medical record system.

The fundamental components of traditional and nontraditional interpretation of lung patterns are very similar. Differences mainly relate to what imaging signs are emphasized as important and choice of terminology. In the nontraditional approach, in lungs with abnormal opacity, the two key signs for prioritizing the differential diagnoses are the degree of lung expansion and the macroscopic distribution of the lung lesion. Additional signs are used, such as the appearance of the opacity, but they are described using terms such as bronchocentric, ground-glass opacity, and consolidation, because they do not indicate a precise histologic classification.

Ultrasound examination of the thorax is an extremely valuable adjunct imaging modality in chest wall, pleural, mediastinal, and pulmonary disease. While air-filled lungs will obscure some deeper pulmonary lesions, ultrasound can evaluate peripheral pulmonary disease, mediastinal masses, and the extent and character of pleural effusions. Ultrasound guidance of needle biopsies and thoracocentesis provides safe and accurate lesion sampling.

Sonographic scanning techniques of the gastrointestinal tract are presented. Normal anatomy and ultrasound appearance of the stomach, small intestine, and large intestine are discussed, followed by the ultrasound appearance of gastrointestinal inflammation, neoplastic disease, and obstruction.

When performing an abdominal ultrasound examination in dogs, a right lateral intercostal approach often is indicated. This approach allows for a complete examination of the abdomen, especially in large deep-chested dogs, dogs with microhepatica, or dogs with a large volume of intestinal gas or peritoneal effusion. The right lateral intercostal approach provides an acoustic window for the evaluation of the right side of the liver, porta hepatis, right limb and body of the pancreas, duodenum, right kidney, right adrenal gland, and hepatic lymph nodes.

CT Diagnosis of Portosystemic Shunts

Allison Zwingenberger

> CT angiography is a new method of diagnosing portal vascular anomalies using volumetric imaging. The scan speed, spatial and contrast resolution, and image display capabilities make CT an excellent tool for depicting anomalous vessels. Normal vessels, congenital intrahepatic and extrahepatic shunts, arterioportal fistulae, and multiple acquired portsosystemic shunts are all readily visible on contrast-enhanced CT images. Technical parameters such as timing, bolus, and respiratory pause are essential to acquiring a diagnostic study.

Scintigraphic Diagnosis of Portosystemic Shunts

Gregory B. Daniel

> Portal scintigraphy is a quick noninvasive method to the diagnosis of portosystemic shunts in dogs and cats. Scintigraphic procedures have evolved over the past 25 years. Currently, trans-splenic portal scintigraphy is the preferred method. High quality studies can be obtained with small radiopharmaceutical doses.

RELATED INTEREST
Veterinary Clinics of North America: Exotic Animal Practice September 2007
(Vol. 10, No. 3)
Neuroanatomy and Neurodiagnostics
Lisa A. Tell, DVM, DAVBP—Avian, and Marguerite F. Knipe, DVM, DACVIM,
Guest Editors

THE CLINICS ARE NOW AVAILABLE ONLINE!

Access your subscription at:
www.theclinics.com

Preface

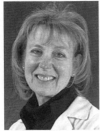 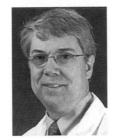

Martha Moon Larson, DVM, MS   Gregory B. Daniel, DVM, MS
Guest Editors

This issue of *Veterinary Clinics of North America: Small Animal Practice* describes new imaging techniques and interpretive methods in the diagnosis of important disease processes. Digital radiography (DR), the subject of the first few articles, has many advantages over film-screen radiography. However, there are important factors to consider before switching to this newer and more expensive technology. The radiographic interpretation of pulmonary disease, whether on DR images, or film-screen systems, has long been a critical, yet challenging, and even intimidating process. Dr. Scrivani's article on an alternative method of looking at pulmonary lung patterns may simplify this process.

Ultrasound is an imaging modality that has been in place in veterinary medicine for many years. However, new uses for this technique continue to be developed. Ultrasound examination of the thorax complements thoracic radiographs and is extremely helpful in the diagnosis of pleural, pulmonary, mediastinal, and chest wall diseases. While gas in the stomach or bowel may preclude complete ultrasound visualization, many important diseases, such as obstruction, neoplasia, and inflammation are easily visualized. The combination of survey abdominal radiographs plus abdominal ultrasound has reduced the need for contrast upper gastrointestinal series in many cases. Ultrasound examination through the right intercostal window allows easier and more complete evaluation of right cranial abdominal anatomy, and is especially helpful in dogs with deep-chested body conformation.

The diagnosis of portosystemic shunts is covered in two articles. Scintigraphic imaging of this disease is often considered the gold standard and is used to reliably rule in or rule out the presence of a shunt. CT angiography is a newer and very detailed imaging modality allowing more exact visualization of abnormal vessels. Surgical treatment of portosystemic shunts is much easier when the exact location of these anomalous vessels is known preoperatively.

Vet Clin Small Anim 39 (2009) ix–x
doi:10.1016/j.cvsm.2009.04.011
0195-5616/09/$ – see front matter © 2009 Elsevier Inc. All rights reserved.

vetsmall.theclinics.com

Thanks to all of the radiologists who contributed their expertise and time to these articles. This issue will hopefully allow us to rethink some of our older diagnostic methods and use newer imaging processes for everyday practice.

Martha Moon Larson, DVM, MS

Gregory B. Daniel, DVM, MS
Department of Small Animal Clinical Sciences
Virginia-Maryland Regional College of Veterinary Medicine
Virginia Tech University
Duckpond Drive, Phase II
Blacksburg, VA 24061, USA

E-mail addresses:
Moonm@vt.edu (M.M. Larson)
Gdaniel@vt.edu (G.B. Daniel)

Digital Imaging

Gregory B. Daniel, DVM, MS

KEYWORDS

- Pixels • Digital matrix • Binary code • Image depth
- Interpolation • File formats • Digital Imaging

Medical imaging is undergoing a revolutionary change. Digital radiographic (DR) image devices are gradually replacing conventional screen film cassettes as radiology departments convert to an all-digital environment. CT and MRI are intrinsically digital. Ultrasound and nuclear medicine images have changed to digital from their film-based ancestors. Radiography is the last modality to make the transition to the digital environment for several reasons. Screen-film combination is a tried and true detector system that produces excellent radiographic images under most circumstances, and, therefore, the motivation for change has been low. Initially, the cost of DR systems was prohibitive, but with advances in computer technology, the cost of these systems continues to drop. Today the cost of conversion to digital in a high-volume department is almost offset by the savings in film, processor maintenance, and film retrieval/archival costs. The large field of view and high spatial resolution requirements of the DR require vast amounts of image data to be stored. Once digital storage space became reasonably priced and wide bandwidth networks became routinely available, DR began to replace film and screens. The convenience and accessibility of digital images are a huge benefit and those who have made the transition indicate that they would not go back.

The modern computer age began in 1971 with the introduction of the Intel 4004 microprocessor.[1] This started the development of relatively inexpensive and reliable computers. In that same decade, the world of computers was combined with medical imaging. The computation power of the microprocessor allowed the EMI Corporation to create the first CT scanner in the 1970s.[2] Mathematically processing the vast number of simultaneous equations required for back projection reconstruction would not be possible without the computer. This was the beginning of the digital era of medical images. Modalities such as CT and MR that require image reconstruction of data were conceived using the microprocessor. The other imaging modalities have converted to digital during the last 15 years. Nuclear medicine was one of the first analog modalities to be converted to the digital age.[3] This was possible because nuclear medicine images contain relatively little information compared with

Department of Small Animal Clinical Sciences, Virginia-Maryland Regional College of Veterinary Medicine, Virginia Tech University, Duckpond Drive, Phase II, Blacksburg, VA 24061, USA
E-mail address: gdaniel@vt.edu

Vet Clin Small Anim 39 (2009) 667–676
doi:10.1016/j.cvsm.2009.04.003
0195-5616/09/$ – see front matter © 2009 Elsevier Inc. All rights reserved.

a radiograph, digital color photograph, or a video. Computer processing of the nuclear medicine images became commonplace in the 1980s, before the advent of powerful computer processors. As computer processors became faster and digital storage became cheaper and more readily available, larger digital images such as radiograph entered into the computer age. Today most radiology departments in human and veterinary teaching hospitals are completely digital. Digital imaging is rapidly expanding into private veterinary practice, and it is inevitable that this trend will continue.

To understand the digital image, we must first review the basic concepts of an image. An image is the visual representation of an object. Images range from simple line drawings to paintings to photographs. The image is a representation of a three-dimensional object on a flat surface, that is, two-dimensional representation. If you isolate a portion of the image to a vertical or horizontal strip, the intensity or color will vary as you look down or across the strip. In isolation, a single strip of the image data is fairly meaningless, but if we combine the strips together, we have an image. The digital image is a two-dimensional array of data with values at each element of the array displayed as an intensity or a color. The array of data is a digital representation of a horizontal or vertical strip of an image. Mathematically, the horizontal strip of the image can be defined as $f(x)$, where f represents the intensity or color at a given location x. The vertical strip of the image can be defined as $f(y)$, where f represents the intensity or color at a given location y. Combining all of the horizontal and vertical strips of data allows us to define the image mathematically as a two-dimensional function.[4]

$$f(x, y)$$

where x and y are the spatial coordinates that identify any location on the image, and the value of f is represented as a color or brightness at the point (x,y).[4] In a digital image, each point of the image and level of brightness are a discrete value.

The two-dimensional array of the digital image is composed of a specific number of rows and columns.[4,5] This two-dimensional array represents a matrix of numbers. Each cell of the matrix has discrete spatial coordinates or a specific address that describes its location on the image. The address of each point can be defined using a Cartesian coordinate system. The Cartesian coordinate system is formed by two perpendicular lines intersecting at the origin. The first coordinate is the *abscissa*, which is the distance from the vertical line, and the *ordinate* is the distance from the horizontal line. The location of the origin (0,0) relative to the image varies with software programs, but for this discussion, let us assume the coordinate at the lower left hand corner of the image is (0,0). The light intensity at each of these points is also given a discrete numerical value. Each address or spatial coordinate is called a picture element or pixel.[6]

Fig. 1 is an image of a canine thorax digitized into discrete picture elements. Note the area of the ninth costrochondral junction located at the spatial coordinates (2230,603). This pixel is 2230 pixels from the left limit of the image and 603 pixels from the bottom of the image. The intensity or the number of counts recorded in this pixel was 176. Using this method, any point of the image could be defined.

MATRIX SIZE

The number of rows and columns (matrix size) will define the spatial resolution of the digital image. The larger the matrix size, the better the resolution of the digital image. (**Fig. 2**) Increasing the matrix size will decrease the size of each pixel. The smallest object represented in the digital image occupies the space of 1 pixel; therefore, the

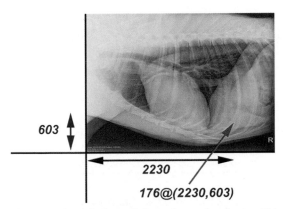

603

2230

176@(2230,603)

Fig. 1. This is a digital image of a right lateral view of a canine thorax. This image was stored into a (2208 x 2668 x 12) matrix, which means the image is 2208 pixels in the vertical direction and 2668 pixels in the horizontal direction. Each pixel has 12 bits of image depth, which means it can store pixel values up to 4096. The pixel at the end of the arrow has a value of 176 and is located 2230 pixels from the y-axis and 603 pixels from the x-axis.

ability to resolve these small objects is dependent on the matrix size of the digital image. These concepts are now familiar to people who have purchased digital cameras. A 7 megapixel camera has better resolution and can resolve smaller objects than a 3 megapixel camera (**Table 1**).

How do you determine what size matrix is needed? The Nyquist theorem defined the minimal matrix size needed to preserve the resolution of the image. This sampling theorem grew out of the field of telecommunications and signal processing and states that any imaging systems should sample at twice the frequency of the objects that you want to resolve. Simply put, if you want to observe two such objects that are the size of a pixel, they must be separated by at least 1 blank pixel.[5,7]

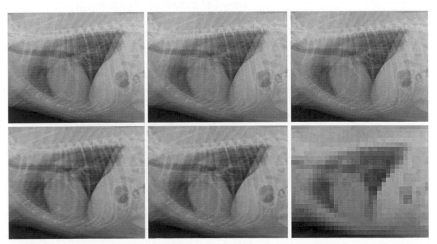

Fig. 2. These are digital images of a right lateral view of a canine thorax. The images are displayed in various matrix sizes ranging from 1600 x 2000 in the upper left to 52 x 63 in the lower right. Note how the size of each individual pixel increases as the matrix size decreases.

Table 1
Common digital matrix sizes for DR and CR images with the corresponding number of pixels within the image

Matrix (Horizontal or x-Axis)	Matrix (Vertical or y-Axis)	Recording Image Size (No. of Pixels)	Mega Pixels
2048	1326	2,715,648	3
2304	1728	3,981,312	4
2560	1920	4,915,200	5
2816	2112	5,947,392	6
3072	2304	7,077,888	7

Many computer displays will enlarge the image without the image looking "pixelly." The process is called image interpolation. This process can partially mask the effect of small matrix size, but resolution is still limited by the digital matrix size of the image. Interpolation, sometimes called resampling, creates new pixels of data and fills in the values based on an extrapolation from the neighboring pixels (**Fig. 3**).

When considering the image quality of an imaging system, one must consider more than just the matrix size of the digital image. Image quality can be limited by the matrix size, that is, pixel limited resolution; however, blurring of the image can occur before it becomes digitalized. For example, a 7 megapixel camera will not produce a sharp image if the lens is not focused on the object. Likewise, a DR system may have a large number of pixels, but if the image capture device is of poor quality, so will be the image.

Spatial resolution of the entire recording system can be measured using an x-ray line pair test phantom (**Fig. 4**). This phantom is composed of lead grid lines separated by equal-size interspaces. The phantom is radiographed and the image evaluated to determine the smallest line pairs that can be seen as separate structures. The spatial resolution is expressed as line pairs per millimeter (lpm) that can be seen using the image system. Direct-exposure film can resolve 50 lpm. Fine-detail screens can resolve 15 lpm. Today, a high-quality digital system can resolve 5 lpm. The unaided eye can resolve 10 lpm. When evaluating DR systems, this resolution factor may be more important than the number of pixels in the image.

Image depth refers to the amount of computer memory assigned to each pixel. Computers store information in a binary code.[6] We are accustomed to working with decimals. This means we count numbers using 10 individual digits (0–9) from which we make up all numbers. Computers are not designed to store Base 10 numbers. It is much easier for computers to register two states, on or off (1 or 0). This is why

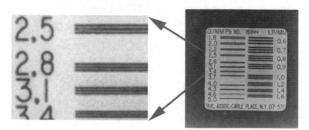

Fig. 3. Image of a line pair phantom showing the number of line pairs per millimeter. The image on the left is an enlargement showing a resolution of the imaging system of 3.1 line pair per mm.

computers use a binary system. Computers store data in discrete storage units called a "bit." Each bit can be either on or off and can be assigned a value of 1 or 0. One bit of computer memory can store two different numbers (0 or 1) using a binary code. It takes 2 bits of computer memory to store up to four different numbers (0 to 3) and so forth (**Table 2**).

The number of bits assigned to the image matrix determines the maximum amount of information that can be stored in an individual pixel. In a black and white image, the number of bits determines the number of shades of gray that can be displayed. The table below shows the relationship between the number of bits and number of shades of gray in a black and white image (**Fig. 5**) (**Table 3**).

Most digital x-ray systems use either 10- or 12-bit images. A 10-bit image contains 1024 shades of gray. A 12-bit image contains 4096 shades of gray. A black and white or grayscale image is considered a single-channel image. A color image will have more than one channel, and when these channels are combined, they are able to displace a variety of colors.[5] For example, a color RBG (red blue green) image has three channels. Each channel will have varying intensities or shades of red, blue, and green, respectively. As such, an RBG image would require three times the amount of computer memory as the same image stored or displayed as a grayscale image. The standard RGB (red green blue) image is 24 bit; each channel has 8 bits, for red, green, and blue. The image is composed of the three-color channels, with each color having brightness intensities between 0 and 255. If the RGB image is 48-bit, each of the three channels will have a 16-bit color scale. Another common type of a digital

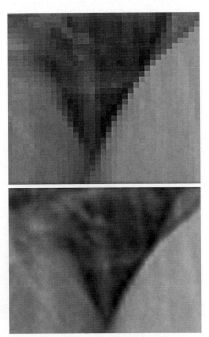

Fig. 4. These are digital images of a right lateral view of a canine thorax, which are enlarged over the area of the caudal vena cava, heart, and diaphragm. The image at the top is displayed with the original pixel size. The image at the bottom has been interpolated into the matrix size of the image display. Note that the pixels are no longer seen, but the image resolution is poor because of the small matrix size the image was stored into.

Table 2
Number of bits required to store whole numbers

Image Depth (Bit)	Binary Number	Base 10 Number
1 bit	0, 1	0, 1
2 bit	10, 11	2, 3
3 bit	100, 101, 110, 111	4, 5, 6, 7
4 bit	1000,1001,1010,1011,1100, 1101,1110,1111	8, 9, 10, 11, 12, 13, 14, 15

color image is the CMYK format. A CMYK image has four channels: cyan, magenta, yellow, and black. The standard CMYK image is 32 bit, made up of four 8-bit channels, one for cyan, one for magenta, one for yellow, and one for black. Because of the multiple channels, color images require much more computer memory to display and store than grayscale images.

A byte is a collection of 8 bits of computer memory. Terms for the number of bytes can be formed using the standard range of SI prefixes as shown below (**Table 4**).

IMAGE DESIGNATION

The designation for a digital image indicates the matrix size and the image depth. A 64 x 64 x 8 designation for an image means the matrix has 64 rows and 64 columns for a total of 4096 pixels. Each pixel has 8 bits of image memory assigned to each, which allows it to store numerical values from 0 to 255. A 256 x 256 x 8 indicates a matrix with 256 rows and 256 columns or 65,536 pixels. Each pixel has 8 bits, which will allow it to store numerical values from 0 to 255. A DR image may have be 2208 x 2668 x 12, which means the matrix has 2208 rows and 2668 columns or 5,890,994 pixels.

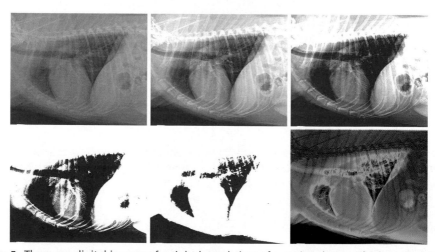

Fig. 5. These are digital images of a right lateral view of a canine thorax. The image on the upper left is displayed in 10-bit image depth using a single-channel grayscale lookup table (1024 shades of gray). The image top center has a 7-bit image depth (128 shades of gray), image top right has a 6-bit image depth (64 shades of gray), the image lower left has a 4 bit (16 shades of gray), and the image lower center has a 1 bit (2 shades of gray). The image on the lower right has an 8-bit, three-channel image using a RBG lookup table.

Table 3
Image depth and the range of numbers and shades of gray that could be stored in the digital image

Image Depth	Range of Base 10 Number	No. of Shades of Gray Displayed in a Black/ White Image	Relationship 2^n Where n = # of Bits of Computer Memory
1 bit	0–1	2	$2^1 = 2$
2 bit	0–3	4	$2^2 = 4$
3 bit	0–8	8	$2^3 = 8$
4 bit	0–15	16	$2^4 = 16$
5 bit	0–31	32	$2^5 = 32$
6 bit	0–63	64	$2^6 = 64$
7 bit	0–127	128	$2^7 = 128$
8 bit	0–255	256	$2^8 = 256$
9 bit	0–511	512	$2^9 = 512$
10 bit	0–1023	1024	$2^{10} = 1024$
12 bit	0–4095	4096	$2^{12} = 4096$

Each pixel has 12 bits of computer memory assigned, which allows up to 4096 shades of gray in each pixel.

DIGITAL IMAGE MEMORY REQUIREMENTS

The product of the total number of pixels in the image and the image depth in bits gives the total amount of computer memory required for displaying or storing each digital image. Image depth (per pixel) x the number of pixels in image matrix = total image size. In addition to the information content of the image, there is nonimage information stored in the file header. The file header information contains data in addition to the digital matrix. The filer header refers to supplemental data placed at the beginning of a block of data being stored. This nonimage information of a medical image contains information about the matrix size, image depth, image acquisition date and time, patient name, medical record number, and so forth. The size of the image header will vary depending on the file format. For the example below, we account for an additional 1024 bytes of storage space for the image header (**Table 5**).

STORAGE DEVICES

Over the years, there has been an evolution of media used to store digital images. Storage media has gotten small, and the storage capacity has greatly increased. Below is a table showing common types of storage media used for digital images (**Table 6**).

Table 4
Prefixes of common units of computer storage capacity

SI Prefix	No. of Bytes
Kilobyte (KB)	1000
Megabyte (MB)	1,000,000
Gigabyte (GB)	1,000,000,000
Terabyte (TB)	1,000,000,000,000

Table 5
Matrix sizes and the corresponding size of the image file

Matrix Size	Image Depth + File Header 1 Byte (8 Bits)	Image Depth + File Header (12 Bits)
64 x 64	4096 + 1024 or 5.1 KB	6144 + 1024 or 7.2 KB
128 x 128	16,384 + 1024 or 17.4 KB	24,576 + 1024 or 25.6 KB
256 x 256	65,536 + 1024 or 66.5 KB	98,304 + 1024 or 99.3 KB
512 x 512	262,144 + 1024 or 263.1 KB	393,216 + 1024 or 394.2 KB
1024 x 1024	1,048,567 + 1024 or 1 MB	1,572,864 + 1024 or 1.6 MB
2208 x 2668[a]	5,890,944 + 1024 or 6 MB	8,836,416 +1024 or 8.8 MB

[a] DR image format

Image file formats are standardized means of organizing and storing images. Because of the need to exchange images between different manufactures of computers, file conversion programs are now commonly found on digital imaging workstations. The subsequent sections describe some common file formats that allow for exchange of images to various computers.

DIGITAL IMAGING AND COMMUNICATIONS IN MEDICINE

The interchange of digital images beyond closed proprietary architectures became important in the 1980s with the development of digital imaging systems (nuclear medicine, CT, MRI, etc) A standardized file exchange protocol was developed by a joint committee between the American College of Radiology and the National Electrical Manufacturers Association[8] (http://medical.nema.org). DICOM is short for Digital Imaging and Communications in Medicine. DICOM defines a communication protocol determining how images and header information are transferred from one computer to another. DICOM differs from other data formats in that it groups information into data sets. This means that a file of a DR actually contains the patient demographic information along with information about equipment used to make the image within the file. The image can never be separated from this information by mistake. All modifications of the file are logged and stored in the DICOM header.

All types of radiology equipment will use DICOM: x-ray, CT, MRI, ultrasound, and nuclear medicine. Images can be sent to a Picture Archival and Communication

Table 6
Comparison of common image storage devices

Media Type	Storage Capacity	No. of Nuclear Medicine Images 256 x 256 x 8	No. of DR Images 2208 x 2668 x 12
5 1/4 in floppy	360 KB	5	0
3 1/2 in diskette	1.44 MB	21	0
Zip drive	250 MB	3814	28
USB drive	2 GB	30,517	226
CD-R	700 MB	10,681	79
DVD	4.7 GB	71,716	531
HD DVD	15 GB (single layer)	225,360	1697

System (PACS) for image comparison or fusion of images such as nuclear medicine scans and radiographs.[9]

Digital images may also be stored as predefined bit maps that are commonly used on personal computer systems. Header information, other than that describing the physical layout of the image, is not included unless it is part of the image bit map. The bit map image format allows the easy transfer and display on computers systems that are not specifically radiology or nuclear medicine computers. Some common Bit map image formats are as follows:

Tagged image file format (TIFF or TIF) is a file format originally created in an attempt to get desktop scanner vendors of the mid-1980s to use the same file format. TIFF is a flexible and adaptable file format that can store images in a wide variety of resolutions, colors, and grayscales. TIFF uses a lossless image compression, which makes it useful for image archiving. The TIFF file format is supported by many systems and is the most commonly used format for scanned images such as photographs.

Joint photographic experts group (JPEG) came from a meeting of a group of photographic experts held in 1982, whose main concern was to work on ways to transmit information. JPEG is now a commonly used image format used by digital cameras. This image file format is used for storage and transmitting images. It provides varying degrees of image compression allowing a selectable trade-off between storage size and image quality. The JPEG format typically achieves 10 to 1 compression with little perceivable loss in image quality. The JPEG compression works best on photographic images. Because of the data loss during compression, these images are not used for quantitative studies.

The graphics interchange format (GIF) is an 8-bit pixel bitmap image format that was introduced by CompuServe in the late 1980s. The file format uses 3 palettes of 256 colors. The color limitation makes the GIF format unsuitable for reproducing color photographs and other images with continuous color, but it is well suited for more simple images such as graphics or logos with solid areas of color. GIF images are commonly used on Webpages due to their wide support and portability.

To display a digital image on a computer monitor, the image must be loaded into the display memory. Every pixel is referred to as an intensity lookup table (LUT) that translates the pixel count value to an intensity or a color value.[6] For a grayscale image, each pixel is assigned a grayscale value from the LUT based on the intensity record by each pixel (see **Fig. 5**). The higher the pixel value, the more intensely the pixel is displayed on the monitor. Images can be displayed as black on a white background (inverse gray) or white on a black background.

The medical grade black and white monitor computers will have 1336 x 2048 pixels (3 megapixel), can display 3061 unique shades of gray, and can cost $4,000 each. A color monitor will have varying intensities of red, green, and blue colors on the monitor. A 24-bit color LUT has 8 bits dedicated to each of the colors, allowing for the display of 256^3 colors or 16 million colors.[1] If red, blue, and green are displayed at their maximum intensity, the color produced is white. If these 3 colors are of equal intensity but less than their maximum intensity, then a shade of gray is displayed. A 24-bit color monitor is able to display 256 shades of gray.

It is inevitable that digital imaging will eventually replace conventional film-based images in radiology and other image-based disciplines. The advantages and disadvantages of digital imaging are discussed in the other articles in this issue. Most of the people who have made the transition to digital imaging would not want to return. The future of diagnostic imaging is good, and digital imaging has created new opportunities and abilities that did not exit a decade before.

REFERENCES

1. Chandra J, March ST, Mukherjee S, et al. Information systems frontiers. Commun ACM 2000;43(1):71–9.
2. Friedland GW, Thurber B. The birth of CT. Am J Roentgenol 1996;176(12):1365–70.
3. Daniel GB. Digital imaging processing. In: Daniel GB, Berry CR, editors. Textbook of veterinary nuclear medicine. 2nd edition. Harrisburg (PA): ACVR; 2006. p. 79–120.
4. Gonzalez R, Wintz P. Digital image processing. London: Mosby; 1977.
5. Russ JC. The image processing handbook. 3rd edition. Boca Raton (FL): CRC Press; 1999.
6. Bushberg JT, Seibert JA, EM L, et al. Computers in medical imaging. In: Bushberg JT, Seibert JA, EM L, et al, editors. The essential physics of medical imaging. Philadelphia: Lippincott Williams & Wilkins; 2002. p. 61–94.
7. Halama J. Representation of gamma camera images by computer. In: Henkin R, Boles M, Dillehay G, editors. Nuclear medicine. St Louis (MO): Mosby; 1996. p. 199–215.
8. Wright MA, Ballance D, Robertson ID, et al. Introduction to DICOM for the practicing veterinarian. Vet Radiol Ultrasound 2008;49(Suppl 1):S14–8.
9. Shiroma JT. An introduction to DICOM. Vet Med 2006;101(Suppl 12):19–20.

Comparing Types of Digital Capture

Laura J. Armbrust, DVM

KEYWORDS

• Digital radiography • Computed radiography • Digital imaging

The availability of digital radiography (DR) equipment to veterinarians is increasing rapidly, and during the past several years, there has been a rapid transition from conventional film-screen radiography to digital systems. Many practitioners are not knowledgeable about the different types of DR equipment. This information becomes especially important when trying to decide what equipment is right for your practice or trying to troubleshoot issues with new equipment. It is also conceivable that film-screen radiographic systems will become obsolete in the not so distant future.[1–5] The different terminology, function, performance, and expense between different DR equipment are highly variable. In addition, as with most technology, there is a rapid change in equipment. The purpose of this article is to provide an up to date synopsis and understanding of the different types of DR equipment.

DIGITAL RADIOGRAPHY EQUIPMENT TERMINOLOGY

In the development of digital imaging systems, the terms "CR," the abbreviation for computed radiography, and "DR," the abbreviation for digital radiography, are commonly used. "DDR" is also used for direct digital radiography, which can be used synonymously with DR. CR systems were first developed by Fuji Medical Corporation in the 1980s with DR products following in the early 1990s.[1–3,5,6] Historically, CR systems use a cassette containing a plate with photostimulable storage phosphor that stores a latent image and is subsequently processed in a plate reader apparatus. (**Fig. 1**) By contrast, DR systems do not use cassettes, but they use a detector that results in the formation of a digital image almost immediately after the exposure is made. (**Fig. 2**) With the rapidly changing technology, there is a large degree of overlap in these classic definitions; therefore, the use of "cassette-based" versus "cassette-less" systems may be easier to understand.[7]

An x-ray generator similar to that used for conventional film-screen radiography is used for both cassette-based and cassette-less digital imaging systems. The aluminum filters and collimator, used to prevent scatter radiation, are similar in DR to those in traditional film-screen radiography. Grids are also used in both cassette-based and

Department of Clinical Sciences, Kansas State University, College of Veterinary Medicine, Veterinary Medical Teaching Hospital, 1800 Denison Avenue, Manhattan, KS 66506, USA
E-mail address: armbrust@vet.ksu.edu

Vet Clin Small Anim 39 (2009) 677–688
doi:10.1016/j.cvsm.2009.04.001
0195-5616/09/$ – see front matter © 2009 Elsevier Inc. All rights reserved.

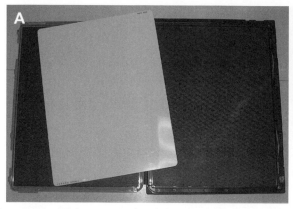
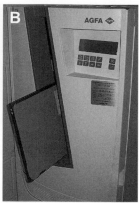

Fig. 1. Image (*A*) is an example of the imaging plate and open cassette for a cassette-based CR system. Image (*B*) shows the cassette being inserted into the plate reader (AGFA CR, AGFA Corp., Greenville, SC).

cassette-less systems; however, digital equipment may require grids with higher grid ratio or higher line pairs per inch. The difference between film-screen systems and digital imaging systems is only the method by which the radiation is detected after the x-rays pass through the patient. Once the images become available for viewing on a computer monitor, the digital systems again become similar, as they result in the same final product[4,5,7] (**Fig. 3**).

CASSETTE-BASED DIGITAL RADIOGRAPHY SYSTEMS

With cassette-based systems (often termed CR), the original radiographic system can still be used, as the only change is the use of a specialized cassette with an imaging plate rather than a cassette containing intensifying screens and film. The imaging plate is coated with photostimulable phosphors (layer of crystals). As x-rays strike the imaging plate, electrons in the crystals are energized to a higher level and stored in electron traps, forming a latent image.[1–7] The exposed "cassette" is placed in a plate reader that extracts the imaging plate from the cassette and scans the plate with a laser light in a series of horizontal lines. During this process, the electrons that

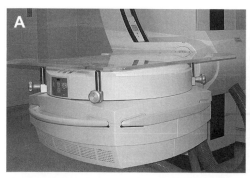
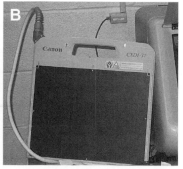

Fig. 2. Two types of cassette-less detectors are shown. (*A*) is a detector used for in-house radiographs (Swissray International, Inc., Elizabeth, NJ). (*B*) is a portable detector (Eklin Medical Systems, Inc., Santa Clara, CA).

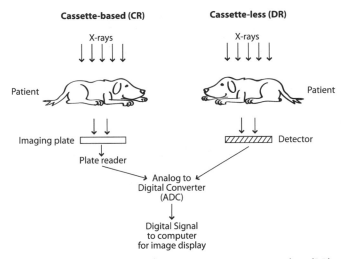

Fig. 3. Schematic of a cassette-based (CR) system versus a cassette-less (DR) system. Both systems are the same as film-screen radiography until the x-rays pass through the patient. The systems become similar again once the electrical (analog) signal is converted to a digital signal. Both types of DR systems result in the same end product, an image viewed on a computer monitor.

were trapped in a higher energy state during x-ray exposure are released into a lower energy state. As the electrons undergo this transition, they stimulate phosphorescence, the emission of visible light. The light that is produced is collected by an optical system coupled to photomultiplier tubes or photodiodes in the reader. The light energy is amplified and converted to an electric signal that is proportional to the light intensity released from the plate. This analog, electrical signal is converted into a digital signal by an analog-to-digital converter. The digital signal is transferred to a computer where the image is displayed. (**Fig. 4**) The imaging plate is then erased by high-intensity white light, replaced in the cassette, and is ready for another exposure.[1–7]

The plate reading time is dependent on the size of the plate, scan speed of the reader, and number of plates that can be processed at any one time (plate readers that process single or multiple plates simultaneously are available). The processing times are generally around 1 to 2 minutes. The imaging plate should be read immediately as the latent image will decay with time.[2,5] The size of the image matrix is

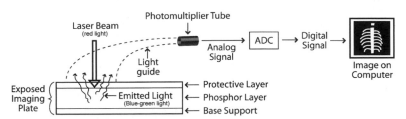

Fig. 4. Schematic of a CR plate being processed inside the plate reader. A laser light results in emission of light from the plate. This light is focused by a light guide and interacts with photomultiplier tubes. The electrical (analog) signal is converted via the analog-to-digital converter to a digital signal that can be displayed on a computer monitor.

a function of the imaging plate dimensions and the pixel sampling pitch. The image size is variable between 8 and 16 MB (megabytes) with a matrix size approximately 2 k by 2.5 k pixels.[7] Imaging plates have differences in spatial resolution and are commonly referred to as standard or high resolution.[4] The standard plates are adequate for general imaging, with the high-resolution plates useful for imaging small parts. Although the high-resolution plates provide better image quality, they are more expensive. Periodic cleaning of plates is necessary, and most manufactures recommend erasing plates at the start of each day/week for maximum image quality. Over time, replacement of cassettes and plates will be needed due to normal wear and tear. Generally, thousands of images can be made before replacement is needed.[1,5]

CASSETTE-LESS DIGITAL RADIOGRAPHY SYSTEMS

For cassetteless digital imaging systems, the image is formed after x-rays expose a detector. Two main categories exist, flat panel and charge coupled device (CCD) detectors. Flat-panel detectors use thin-film transistor (TFT) technology.[4–8] The TFT arrays are composed of many small detector elements. When the x-rays expose a TFT, the energy is converted to an electrical charge. There are two main ways this conversion from x-ray energy to electrical charge occurs, direct and indirect. Indirect detectors convert the x-ray energy into light via a scintillator (commonly cesium iodide crystals). The light is converted to an electrical signal via a photodiode arrays (commonly amorphous silicon). Direct detectors convert the x-ray energy directly into an electrical pulse via a photoconductive layer (such as amorphous selenium) linked directly to the TFT (**Fig. 5**).

Systems based on CCD technology are also becoming more widely available. CCD systems are considered a type of indirect conversion, because a scintillator is used to convert x-ray energy to light.[4–8] An optical coupling device minifies the light beam to the small dimension of a CCD chip. The light energy is converted to an electrical signal that is sent to the computer (**Fig. 6**).

The flat panel and CCD detectors are built directly into the table or are portable (flat panel only), so there is no use of cassettes. The information is immediately transferred to a computer. Since these systems are independent of any cassette or reader/processor, they result in faster image generation, within seconds of exposure. In

Flat Panel - Thin Film Transistor

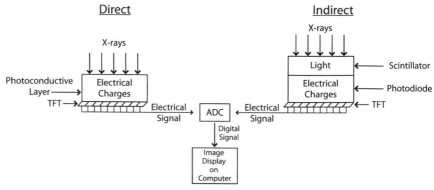

Fig. 5. Schematic of a direct and indirect cassette-less (DR) system. The indirect system requires an extra step of x-ray to light conversion.

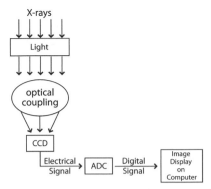

Fig. 6. Schematic of a CCD indirect digital detector. The x-rays strike a scintillator material that produces light. The light is then focused via an optical coupling device before reaching the CCD. As with other types of digital systems, this analog (electrical) signal is converted to a digital signal for display.

general, flat-panel detectors are more expensive than CCD. CCD detectors often have decreased image quality due to a lower signal-to-noise ratio. CCD detectors are not portable and horizontal, or cross-beam imaging is not possible.[5,8] **Table 1** lists comparisons between detectors.

Some vendors use entirely new radiographic systems for the transition to cassette-less systems, whereas other vendors can retrofit existing x-ray tables to allow for insertion of the digital detectors.[1,6,7,9] Although there is no cleaning and erasure process required as with imaging plates, the digital detectors need correction/

Table 1
Comparison of traditional film-screen radiography, cassette-based, and cassette-less digital radiography system.

	Film-Screen	Cassette-Based CR	Cassette-Less Flat-Panel direct	Cassette-Less Flat-Panel Indirect	Cassette-Less CCD Indirect
Startup cost	Low	Moderate	High	High	Moderate
Integration with current equipment	Yes	Yes	Possible	Possible	Possible
Throughput	Low	Low	High	High	High
Latitude	Low	Moderate to high	Moderate to high	Moderate to high	Moderate
Spatial resolution	High	Moderate	Moderate	Moderate	Moderate
Contrast resolution	Low	High	High	High	High
DQE (detector efficiency)	Low	Moderate	High	High	Moderate
Ability to postprocess	No	Yes	Yes	Yes	Yes
Portable	Yes	Yes	Yes	Yes	No
Image quality	Moderate	High	High	High	Moderate

Data from Widmer WR. Acquisition hardware for digital imaging. Vet Radiol Ultrasound 2008;49(1 Supp 1):S2–8; and Digital x-ray systems. Part 1: an introduction to DX technologies and an evaluation of cassette DX systems. Health Devices 2001;30(8):273.

calibration performed on a regular basis. This calibration process is highly variable dependent on the type of detector and manufacturer. If calibration is not performed, then noise artifacts and nonfunctioning pixels will degrade image quality.[6–8]

IMAGE PROCESSING, DISPLAY, AND QUALITY COMPARISONS

In addition to understanding the functional differences between DR systems, one must also be able to evaluate and compare the final image product between vendors. Factors that vary among digital systems include detective quantum efficiency (DQE—the efficiency of the detector for identifying incident X-ray photons), dynamic range, spatial sampling, spatial resolution, noise, and contrast resolution[8,10] (see **Table 1**). Some of these are listed as part of the product specifications, whereas others are more difficult to evaluate. The company-specific software programs vary, and companies may include certain hardware, whereas other hardware must be purchased separately. The vendor-specific software programs create a grayscale level for each pixel. The raw image data can be adjusted for under- or overexposure before display. The specific algorithms vary between digital systems and define multiple factors such as contrast resolution, optical density, contrast type (linear or nonlinear), spatial and frequency resolution, and the degree of edge enhancement.[1,2,5,11] The user can then further manipulate the image via postprocessing steps. The minimum standard display controls should include window and level (analogous to contrast and brightness), pan, zoom, flip, rotate, and measuring tools.[5,7,10,11] Most programs have many additional features to enhance diagnostic utility. The ability to vary the image contrast and brightness is very useful for evaluating both the soft tissue and bone on the same image (**Fig. 7**).

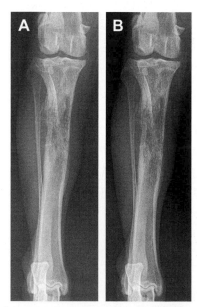

Fig. 7. The digital image of the tibia is windowed and leveled for viewing the soft tissues in (*A*) and for bone viewing in (*B*). Notice that in (*A*) there is increased brightness and wider latitude (*many shades of gray*). In (*B*) the background is darker and the image is of higher contrast (*more black and white*).

The computer hardware with DR systems includes a user interface, or quality control workstation, to enter and link the patient information with the digital image and to review the digital images before final acceptance (**Fig. 8**). Consideration should be given to the quality of the computer monitor not only at the quality control workstation but also most importantly at the monitors that are used for the final interpretation. Monitor size, resolution, brightness (luminance), and contrast should all be considered.[7,10,12] These interpretation stations may come as part of the overall package or may require additional purchase, which can be costly. The recommended guidelines for interpretation workstations include the use of grayscale liquid crystal display monitors with a ratio of maximum luminance to the minimum luminance of at least 50 or at least 250 cd (candela)/m^2. The monitor should be at minimum 2 MP (megapixal) with a contrast ratio of 600:1 to 1000:1 for diagnostic viewing.[7,10] High-quality color monitors have also recently performed well for imaging viewing.[13] To maximize interpretation, an antiglare coating is useful, and ambient light should be kept to a minimum. Often multiple monitors are used in combination so that multiple views of the same patient can be evaluated simultaneously (**Fig. 9**). Standard computer monitors do provide high enough quality to use for reviewing DRs with clients. Consider the number of workstations and monitors that will be required in your particular practice setting when determining the final cost.

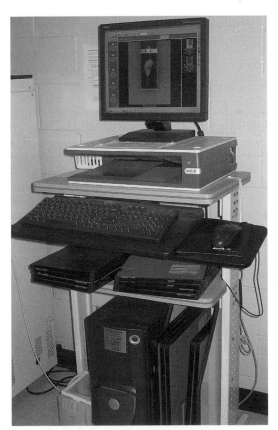

Fig. 8. An example of a quality control workstation (AGFA CR, AGFA Corp., Greenville, SC), where patient data can be entered and the radiographs approved for quality before sending on to the interpretation station and other locations.

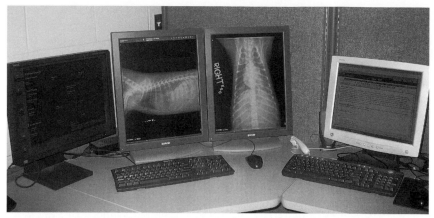

Fig. 9. An example of an interpretation work area with two interpretation monitors (3 megapixel) and two ancillary monitors for reviewing patient information and dictation.

Before a purchasing decision is made, images from various vendors should be compared and on-site visits, where equipment is installed and functioning, can be very useful. Remember that there are many steps to the process, and the final product will be only as good as the rate-limiting step.

ADVANTAGES AND DISADVANTAGES OF DIGITAL RADIOGRAPHY EQUIPMENT

Conventional film-screen radiography has many limitations compared with DR. The limitations for film-screen include narrow exposure latitude (there is little room for exposure error to obtain a diagnostic film), the need for chemical processing, dark room maintenance, incompatibility with electronic transmission and image enhancement, loss of films, deterioration of films over time, film storage space, and high costs for film materials and labor.[1-7] Conversely, DR allows for convenience of digital image format, storage in a much smaller space, quick access for later reference, lower film cost, less staff required for archiving, elimination of processor and chemicals, fewer repeat exposures, rapid image acquisition, which increases throughput, and remote image interpretation (teleradiology) (see **Table 1**).[1-8,10-12]

Although the spatial resolution of DR systems, 2.5 to 5 lpm (line pairs/mm), does not match up to conventional film-screen (2.5–15 lpm), new technology is getting closer everyday. The improved contrast resolution and latitude seen with digital systems more than overcome this limitation.[4,5] In fact, image contrast and latitude are one of the major advantages of DR over traditional film-screen systems. Latitude, also termed dynamic range, is the range of exposures that will result in a useable, or diagnostic, image. The latitude of DR is much greater than that of film-screen systems.[1-3,6,12] Film-screen systems typically have either good latitude or good contrast, but not both. Once a film is exposed and processed, there is no way to adjust the image contrast or blackness. Digital images can be adjusted to display high-contrast (few shades of gray) or wide latitude (many shades of gray) (**Fig. 10**).

Another major advantage of DR systems is the wide range of exposure factors that can be used without compromising the diagnostic value of the image.[1,2,6] Thus, over- and underexposure problems that are so common when using a film-based system are much less problematic in the digital environment.

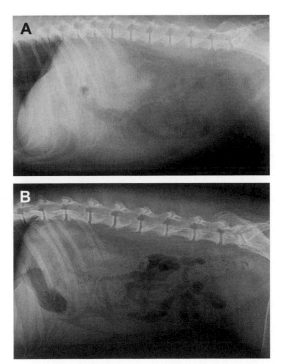

Fig. 10. A conventional film-screen radiograph (*A*) that has a wide latitude but poor contrast compared with a digital radiograph (*B*) that exhibits both wide latitude and excellent contrast.

Some vendors list decreased exposure to staff and patients as an advantage of DR. This may be true if the incidence of repeat radiographs decreases; however, the exposure technique for most DR systems are roughly comparable to exposures used with 200-speed film-screen systems.[3] In addition, processing errors that can render an excellent-quality radiograph nondiagnostic are not issues in DR, as the images are processed electronically using a computer rather than physically in the darkroom. Some artifacts can be seen during digital processing.

Another major limitation of DR is the higher initial investment, especially with cassette-less systems. Lack of familiarity with acquiring digital images and interpretation of digital images must also be accounted for. The technology that is required and networking the systems to make them useful are complicated.

ADDITIONAL TYPES OF DIGITAL CAPTURE

Handheld digital cameras and film digitizers can be used to convert film-based images into a digital format.[12,14] The disadvantage of these methods are the introduction of noise and limited grayscale (dynamic) range.[7,12] The file type produced and amount of image compression are variable and can lead to poor-quality digital images. Many teleradiology services will not accept images produced by these methods. Although these methods are not recommended, information exists describing how to maximize image quality.[12,15]

CONSIDERATIONS FOR PURCHASE

Although an all-inclusive list is almost impossible to create, researching the following is a good place to start when comparing DR systems:

1. Economically justifiable:
   A. Capital costs
   B. Maintenance/service costs/warranty
   C. Intangible costs such as time for processing images, quality control, and user maintenance
2. Make sure you understand what type of system you are purchasing (cassette-based, cassetteless, hybrid)—in general terms of cost, you often get what you pay for
3. If a cassette-less system is used, what type and how often is detector calibration required?
4. For cassette-based systems what is the longevity of the cassette and plate? How many plates come with the initial purchase?
5. Positioning flexibility/portability
6. Ease of use
7. Patient throughput
8. Company stability—Will the company be in business to service and upgrade equipment in the future?
9. Service—own service or outsourced, up-time guarantee, loaners available
10. Built-in system redundancy—What happens when the system goes down?
11. Application support—training, hours, accessibility
12. Expandability—add on features and hardware and software upgrades
13. Workflow—does it tie in with your current hospital management system?
14. Uses—in house or mobile?
15. Teleradiology availability
16. Evaluate image quality
    A. Zoom the image—more readily displays the noise
    B. Compare images on the same monitor
    C. Evaluate both small parts and large patients
    D. Look for the halo artifact around implants

Remember that any digital imaging system is only as good as its weakest link.

SUMMARY

A multitude of DR systems are available. These systems can be both cassette-based (CR) or cassette-less (DR). An understanding of the differences between the digital systems and film-screen radiography is needed to purchase systems and get the most benefit out of your current system. Comparisons between systems are summarized in **Table 1**.

DR COMPANIES (LIST IS NOT ALL INCLUSIVE AND IS PROVIDED ALPHABETICALLY) WEBSITES WERE ACCESSED AUGUST 2008:

1. AFP Veterinary Digital Systems- http://www.afpimaging.com/digivet.
2. AGFA- http://www.agfa.com/en/he/solutions/radiology/digital_x_ray/index.jsp.
3. AllPro Imaging- http://www.allproimaging.com/Veterinary/default.aspx.
4. Canon- http://medical.canon-europe.com/X-Ray/index.asp.

5. Del Medical- http://www.delmedical.com/cgi-bin/r.cgi/b_productdetail.html? SESSION=E6XpqlJzNz&ProductID=52.
6. Eklin- http://www.eklin.com/.
7. Fuji- http://www.fujimed.com/products-services/imaging-systems/digital-xray/ default.asp?location=1&area=10&id=0&subid=0.
8. iCRco- http://www.icrcompany.com/.
9. IDEXX- http://www.idexx.com/.
10. InnoVet- http://www.innovet4vets.com/innovet_home.html.
11. Kodak- http://www.kodakdental.com/en/digitalImaging/index.html?pID=2154.
12. Konica- http://www.konicaminolta.com/medicalusa/.
13. Medicatech- http://www.medicatechusa.com/.
14. Phillips- http://www.medical.philips.com/main/products/xray/products/radiography/ digital/index.html.
15. Quantum Medical Imaging- http://www.quantummedical.net/.
16. Sedecal- http://www.tallentxray.com/sedecal_VET_xray.html.
17. Siemens-   http://www.medical.siemens.com/webapp/wcs/stores/servlet/ CategoryDisplay~q_catalogId~e_-1~a_categoryId~e_14,1,001.htm,007,010, 14,100,283,283~a_catTree~e_12,660~a_langId~e_-1~a_storeId~e_10,759.
18. Sound Technologies-DR; http://www.soundvet.com/
19. Swissray- http://www.swissray.com/.
20. Universal; http://www.universalultrasound.com/productpages/digitalradiography. htm.

ACKNOWLEDGMENTS

The author acknowledges Mal Hoover for her contribution to **Figs. 3–6**.

REFERENCES

1. Mattoon JS, Smith C. Breakthroughs in radiography. Computed radiography. Compendium 2004;17(1):58–66.
2. Roberts GD, Graham JP. Computed radiography. In: Kraft SL, Roberts GD, editors. Modern diagnostic imaging, veterinary clinics of North America. Equine practice. Philadelphia: WB Saunders; 2001. p. 47–61.
3. Stearns ED. Computed radiography in perspective. National Association of Veterinary Technicians in America Journal 2004;53–8.
4. Bansal GJ. Digital radiography. A comparison with modern conventional imaging. Postgrad Med J 2006;82:425–8.
5. Widmer WR. Acquisition hardware for digital imaging. Vet Radiol Ultrasound 2008;49(1 Supp 1):S2–8.
6. Digital x-ray systems. Part 1: an introduction to DX technologies and an evaluation of cassette DX systems. Health Devices 2001;30(8):273–84.
7. American College of Radiology. American college of radiology practice guideline. Available at: http://www.acr.org/SecondaryMainMenuCategories/quality_safety/ guidelines/dx/digital_radiography.aspx.
8. Seibert JA. The digital capture question. A comparison of digital detectors. Available at: http://www.imagingeconomics.com/issues/articles/2003-06_04.asp. Accessed August 21, 2008.
9. Bushberg JT, Seibert JA, Leidholdt EM, et al. Computers in medical imaging. In: Passano WM, editor. The essential physics of medical imaging. Maryland: Williams & Wilkins; 1994.
10. Puchalski SM. Image display. Vet Radiol Ultrasound 2008;49(1 Supp 1):S9–13.

11. Lo WY, Puchalski SM. Digital image processing. Vet Radiol Ultrasound 2008; 49(1 Supp 1):S42–7.

12. Papageorges M. Image capture devices. In: Papageorges M, editor. Understanding and using telemedicine: how to harness the telecommunication revolution. Clackamas: Veterinary Diagnostic Imaging and Cytopathology Publishing, Inc. 1999.

13. Krupinski EA, Roehrig H, Fan J, et al. Monochrome versus color softcopy displays for teleradiology: observer performance and visual search efficiency. Telemed J E Health 2007;13(6):675–81.

14. Sistrom CL, Gray SB. Digital cameras for reproducing radiologic images: evaluation of three cameras. AJR Am J Roentgenol 1998;170:279–84.

15. Whitehouse RW. Use of digital cameras for radiographs: how to get the best pictures. J R Soc Med 1999;92:178–82.

Digital Radiographic Artifacts

David A. Jiménez, DVM*, Laura J. Armbrust, DVM

KEYWORDS

- Artifact • Digital • Computed • Radiographic
- Digital radiography • Computed radiography
- Image • Error

Digital radiographic systems used in veterinary medicine include photostimulable phosphor systems, indirect digital radiography, and direct digital radiography. Photostimulable phosphor systems are usually cassette-based and are commonly referred to as computed radiography (CR). Indirect and direct digital radiography are usually cassetteless and are commonly referred to as digital radiography (DR). Given the development of equipment that incorporates features common to both DR and CR, the terms *cassette-based* and *cassetteless* may be a more appropriate means to classify digital imaging systems.[1,2]

Digital systems are being used in an increasing number of veterinary hospitals and differs substantially from film-screen (FS) radiography. Although some artifacts seen with FS appear similar to those created by CR and DR, several unique artifacts can be seen with digital systems. Artifacts in radiography can be detrimental to interpretation by decreasing visualization or altering the appearance of an area of interest. Understanding the cause of artifacts and method of resolution is paramount in acquiring high-quality digital images.

A digital artifact can be categorized according to the step during which it was created. The major categories are preexposure, exposure, postexposure, reading, and workstation artifacts (**Tables 1** and **2**). Identifying the step during which an artifact was created is important in correcting the error and minimizing its occurrence in future studies. Hardware and software troubleshooting of digital artifacts differs from methods used for FS.

The purpose of this article is to help categorize and describe artifacts encountered when using DR and CR. Understanding how digital radiographs are created is necessary for isolating a cause and reducing the occurrence of digital artifacts.

PREEXPOSURE ARTIFACTS
Storage Scatter

Artifacts due to exposure from extraneous radiation sources may occur at any time before an imaging plate reading when using CR.[3] Imaging plates are more sensitive

Department of Clinical Sciences, Kansas State University, College of Veterinary Medicine, Veterinary Medical Teaching Hospital, 1800 Denison Avenue, Manhattan, KS 66506, USA
* Corresponding author.
E-mail address: djimenez@vet.k-state.edu (D.A. Jiménez).

Table 1
Artifacts created with cassette-based computed radiography

Category	Artifact
Preexposure	Storage scatter
	Cracks
	Partial erasure
	Phantom image
Exposure	Upside-down cassette
	Backscatter
	Grid cutoff
	Double exposure
	Quantum mottle
	Saturation
Postexposure	Light leak
	Fading
Reading	Debris
	Dirty light guide
	Skipped scan lines
	Moiré
Workstation	Faulty transfer
	Border detection
	Diagnostic specifier
	Clipping
	Density threshold
	Überschwinger

to radiation when compared with conventional film and, therefore, may be more noticeably affected.[4–6] Extraneous radiation exposure may be from background radiation or scatter produced during diagnostic imaging studies. Uneven distribution of radiation exposure or attenuation pattern of radiation on the imaging plate may result in a noticeable pattern on the image (**Table 3**).[7] A distinct pattern has been produced from shelving units and image plate holders located between the radiation source and the plate. Evenly distributed scatter radiation will result in a generalized increase in exposure and darkening of the image due to fogging. To avoid exposure by extraneous or scatter radiation, do not store CR image plates within the radiology suite. Exposure to background radiation may accumulate over time. Erasure of imaging plates is recommended before use and is often performed at the beginning of each workday.[3]

Cracks

During the reading process, imaging plates are removed from the cassette and transported through the reader. There is the potential of physical damage to the imaging plate during this process. Damage to the imaging plate can also occur while handling the imaging plate during routine maintenance and cleaning.[8] Cracks in the imaging plate create linear or focal white artifacts (**Table 4**). These cracks are more likely to occur in the periphery and, therefore, only infrequently superimpose over the area of interest.[3,7,9,10] Cracks located more centrally may be misinterpreted as foreign material or osseous fragments.[9] Imaging plates with higher inherent resolution may be more susceptible to cracks due to their thin phosphor layer, thin surface protective layer, and small phosphor size.[7] Proper maintenance of the imaging plate, cassette,

Table 2
Artifacts created with cassette-less digital radiography

Category	Artifact
Preexposure	Memory Dead pixels Calibration mask
Exposure	Grid cutoff Double exposure Quantum mottle Saturation Paradoxic overexposure effect Planking Radiofrequency interference
Reading	Moiré
Workstation	Faulty transfer Border detection Diagnostic specifier Clipping Density threshold Überschwinger

and imaging plate reader may reduce the occurrence of cracks and their associated artifacts. It is recommended to wear cotton gloves when gingerly handling imaging plates. Follow the manufacturer's suggestions for cleaning. Imaging plates with cracks detrimental to interpretation should be replaced.[10]

Partial Erasure

Incomplete erasure of CR imaging plates may result in retention of the previous image. During the reading process, a red laser scans the imaging plate to release the latent image in the form of a green light. This process does not release all the energy stored

Table 3
Artifacts with decreased overall image quality

Artifact	Category	Cause	Remedy
Storage scatter	Preexposure	Exposure to scatter and background radiation	Erase imaging plates before use Protect from scatter radiation
Dead pixels	Preexposure	Nonfunctional detector elements Focal blurring techniques	Map and cancel out dead pixels Replace detector array as needed
Quantum mottle	Exposure	Decreased number of incident x-rays	Increase exposure technique
Fading	Postexposure	Excessive time between exposure and reading	Read imaging plates shortly after exposure
Diagnostic specifier	Workstation	Incorrect selection of region of interest	Choose correct region of interest for each study

Table 4
Artifacts with white dots or lines

Artifact	Category	Cause	Remedy
Cracks	Preexposure	Physical damage to imaging plate	Handle imaging plates carefully Replace imaging plates as needed
Upside-down cassette	Exposure	Incorrect cassette orientation during exposure	Ensure correct cassette orientation before use
Debris	Reading	Debris on imaging plate blocks emission of light	Clean imaging plates routinely and as needed
Dirty light guide	Reading	Dirt on the light guide blocks transmission of light	Clean the light guide routinely and as needed

within the imaging plate. For complete erasure, the imaging plate is usually exposed to bright white light.[11] Errors in complete erasure may occur due to erasure light malfunction. Burnt out, dirty, or fading light bulbs may create insufficient amounts of white light.[12] Alternatively, overexposure of the imaging plate increases the amount of stored energy and makes incomplete release of energy more likely. Release of stored energy is also more difficult with newer, more stable imaging plates.[7] If erasure is incomplete, it appears as a faint superimposition of the previous image over the more recent image (**Table 5**).[3] To avoid partial erasure artifacts, erasure lights should be cleaned and replaced as needed. Some systems incorporate an additional exposure to ultraviolet (UV) light for more efficient erasure.[7]

Phantom Image

Phantom image artifacts may be seen with CR. After appropriate image plate erasure, a latent image is not immediately detectable. Should the imaging plate remain unused for a prolonged period of time, the previous latent image may become detectable

Table 5
Artifacts with double images

Artifact	Category	Cause	Remedy
Partial erasure	Preexposure	Erasure light failure	Replace erasure light bulbs as needed Erase with additional UV light
Phantom image	Preexposure	Excessive time between erasure and exposure	Erase imaging plates before use
Memory	Preexposure	Retained charge in detector	Ground conductive layers Wait in between radiographs
Double exposure	Exposure	Multiple radiographs taken with a single imaging plate Memory or transfer errors	Read imaging plates after each use Use reliable power supply and data transfer

again.[10] This usually requires several days or longer to occur but may depend on specific imaging plate characteristics and erasure methods.[12] When the imaging plate is subsequently used, the previous image appears faintly superimposed over the more recent image (see **Table 5**). To avoid phantom image artifact, it is recommended that imaging plates be erased before use. This is usually performed at the beginning of each workday.[9,10]

Memory

Photodiodes used with indirect DR undergo excitation when they convert fluorescent light into an electrical charge.[2] Photoconductors used with direct DR undergo excitation when exposed to x-rays.[11] This is an integral process in creating an electrical impulse, which is temporarily stored by the detector array in the form of a latent image.[11] After detector array discharge and image read-out, a brief period of time is required for photodiodes and photoconductors to return to their ground state. If a radiograph is acquired during this short recovery period, the pattern of residual excitation may superimpose over the following radiograph (see **Table 5**).[13] Negative memory artifacts have been seen with indirect DR and exhibit grayscale reversal of the faint, summated prior radiograph (**Fig. 1**).[14] Positive memory artifacts have been seen with direct DR using a selenium-based photoconductor.[13] They appear as a faint summation of the previous image. Proper grounding of the molecularly excitable layers of DR equipment is usually applied immediately before exposure to reduce electrical inhomogeneities.[2] Functional electrical conduction and grounding should decrease the occurrence of memory artifacts. If necessary, a brief delay between one radiograph and the next will reduce this artifact.

Dead Pixels

Detector arrays used with DR are comprised of rows and columns of detector elements that correspond to each pixel on the radiograph. When manufactured, a small fraction of detector elements is nonfunctional and referred to as dead pixels (see **Table 3**).[11] The detector array is calibrated and mapped for dead pixels. Values for dead pixels are interpolated from the values of adjacent pixels.[15,16] This method of compensation may be problematic when dead pixels are juxtaposed.[16] With use, progressively more detector elements may fail.[15] Dead pixel artifacts appear as white or black spots on a radiograph.[15] Detector array mapping and postprocessing

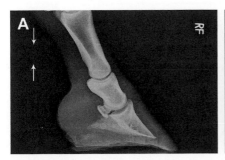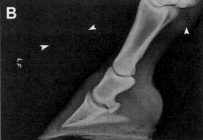

Fig. 1. Lateromedial radiographs of the right and left front feet of a horse, using indirect DR. The radiograph of the right front foot (*A*) has multiple rectangular areas of variable shades of gray (*in between white arrows*) due to planking artifact. The radiograph of the left foot (*B*) was taken shortly afterward. It displays planking artifact and memory artifact. The silhouette of the previous right front foot and marker is superimposed over the image (*white arrowheads*).

techniques can be modified multiple times throughout the life of the detector array to account for additional detector element failure.[15,16] When an excessive percentage of detector elements do not function, the overall image quality is decreased. Detector arrays should be replaced as needed.

Calibration Mask

X-ray fields are not uniform within the field of view or among radiographic equipment. Furthermore, there are inherent differences in signal amplification and sensitivity throughout the surface of a detector array. Each DR system is tested to detect nonuniformity and apply a calibration mask, which compensates for inhomogeneities. In the absence of an object, x-ray exposure of a calibrated detector should result in a uniformly gray image. Errors in calibration may become visible on each radiograph acquired afterward (**Table 6**). Attenuation of x-rays by debris or radiographic contrast medium during the calibration process will be imprinted on the mask and appear as dark silhouettes of the material on future studies (**Fig. 2**).[14] If a border of the detector array is outside of the x-ray field during calibration, the mask will severely darken the periphery of subsequent radiographs.[14] Irregularities of a table in a nonstationary setup may be in a different position during calibration and clinical use. These irregularities can appear as a negative image superimposed over the patient study.[14] Areas of the table with increased attenuation during calibration appear darker on future studies, and areas of decreased attenuation appear lighter. Debris or contrast medium in the tube housing or on the collimator window during calibration will have a similar effect but appear magnified and blurred due to x-ray beam geometry.[14] Cleaning all equipment and placing detectors on the tabletop, if possible, can decrease artifacts associated with calibration.

Table 6
Artifacts with image derangement and variable shades of gray

Artifact	Category	Cause	Remedy
Calibration mask	Preexposure	Variable attenuation during calibration	Clean equipment and recalibrate Use table-top technique for calibration
Planking	Exposure	Variable amplification of separate array sections	Calibrate equipment routinely and as needed Decrease exposure technique as needed
RF interference	Exposure	RF affecting detector	Avoid RF sources Maintain proper RF shielding
Skipped scan lines	Reading	Jarring active imaging reader Power fluctuation	Avoid abrupt contact with imaging plate reader when in use Provide stable power supply
Faulty transfer	Workstation	Loose data cable Power fluctuation Memory error	Use reliable method of data transfer Provide stable power supply Replace software as needed

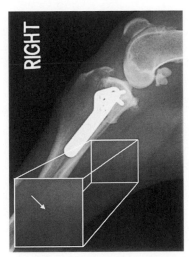

Fig. 2. Mediolateral radiograph of the right stifle of a dog, using direct DR. Multiple dark spots were present at the same location on every radiograph taken after calibration of the direct DR detector. The dark spots present over the gastrocnemius muscle of the patient (*arrow*) are representative of the repeatable calibration mask artifacts seen.

EXPOSURE ARTIFACTS
Upside-down Cassette

Errors in cassette orientation can occur with CR and are similar to those described with FS. Cassette construction differs between manufacturers. An important difference lies in the presence or absence of lead foil lining the back of the cassette. When a radiograph is acquired with the cassette oriented upside down, the x-rays pass through the back of the cassette before being incident on the imaging plate (see **Table 4**). The construction of the back of the cassette will attenuate x-rays and may be seen as a representative underexposed pattern superimposed over the patient (**Fig. 3**).[3,9] When using cassettes with lead backing, a large amount of more uniform attenuation may result in a completely white or severely underexposed image. Ensuring correct orientation of the cassette during each radiographic exposure will help in avoiding artifacts associated with upside-down cassettes.

Backscatter

X-rays that pass through the front of the cassette, imaging plate, and back of the cassette can create scatter radiation as they strike distal objects. Scatter disperses in multiple directions and may return toward the CR cassette. This can increase imaging plate exposure to scatter radiation in a diffuse or nonuniform pattern (**Table 7**). Nonuniform scatter exposure can be due to the shape of the backscattering object or construction of the back of the cassette. A larger amount of backscatter and increased exposure may be present in the periphery of the radiograph.[14] Increased amounts of backscatter can be created with a high kVp technique, large field of view, and increased object thickness.[4,5] Backscatter is most noticeable when a gap is present between the backscattering object and cassette.[5] The imaging plates used with CR are more sensitive to x-ray exposure than film-screen combinations.[4,5,7,9] The amount of x-ray transmission through the back of the cassette can be largely decreased by a lead foil lining. This same lining will attenuate scatter radiation, including backscatter, from inadvertently exposing the imaging plate.

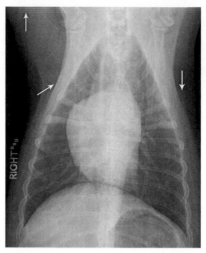

Fig. 3. Ventrodorsal thoracic radiograph of a dog, using CR. The cassette was placed upside down. X-rays were partially attenuated by the back of the cassette before being incident on the imaging plate. The cassette back construction appears as white lines and circles (*white arrows*) superimposed over the image.

Grid Cutoff

Focused grids are used to decrease scatter radiation from reaching the imaging plate or detector. They are composed of low-density material separated by parallel lead strips that are angled toward the x-ray tube. Grids are recommended to be used with most DR and CR studies.[9] Incorrect positioning or orientation of the grid may lead to excessive reduction of incident x-rays by the lead strips in a manner similar

Table 7 Artifacts with darker areas			
Artifact	**Category**	**Cause**	**Remedy**
Backscatter	Exposure	Scattering from objects below the cassette	Use cassettes with lead backing
		High exposure settings	Decrease exposure technique as needed
Saturation	Exposure	Exceeding maximal detectable exposure	Reduce exposure technique
Border detection	Workstation	Radiograph including high-density objects	Use lower level of automated border detection
		Misaligned cassette and field of view	Align the cassette with the field of view
			Center the area of interest
Density threshold	Workstation	High-density objects included in image analysis	Set upper limit on densities included in image analysis
Clipping	Workstation	Decreased image file size	Modify processing to include all pertinent data

to that described for FS (**Table 8**).[11] The increased sensitivity of DR equipment and ability to manipulate the image can make uniform alterations in x-ray attenuation less detrimental to overall image quality. Increased uniform attenuation may be seen when there is angulation or decentering of the grid. DR systems dedicated to an imaging table may have a removable grid. Incorrect placement of a focused grid in an upside-down orientation will lead to nonuniform attenuation of x-rays. The central area of the radiograph will be minimally affected, and attenuation will be increasingly more severe toward the periphery of the image. This may appear as underexposed, white stripes on either edge of the radiograph (**Fig. 4**).[12] This artifact can be avoided by checking for correct grid placement before exposure.

Double Exposure

CR plates may be mistakenly used for multiple exposures or studies without being read or erased between each one.[4,7,14,17] The radiograph will then appear as 2 images summated on each other (**Fig. 5**) (see **Table 5**). This can also occur with FS and results in double images, which are consequently overexposed. In contrast, the larger latitude of CR allows for double exposures to have a seemingly normal overall opacity.[14] The opacity of each of the summated exposures relative to each other depends on the difference in the technique used for each one.[4,7] Double exposures have also been observed using DR as a result of electrical interruptions or data transfer error.[12] Double exposures can be avoided by reading each imaging plate immediately after its exposure. When using DR, scheduled maintenance and use of stable data transfer will reduce double-exposure artifact.

Quantum Mottle

All images created using CR or DR contain a certain amount of noise. This is mostly due to the fluctuations in the number of x-ray photons throughout the image, called quantum mottle (see **Table 3**).[1] The prominence of quantum mottle is dependent on the amount of data representing the object of interest in proportion to the amount of noise. This relationship is referred to as the signal-to-noise ratio (SNR). The SNR increases when the number of x-rays incident on the imaging plate or detector increases. The use of low mAs techniques or increased attenuation of the primary x-ray beam may result in an insufficient number of incident x-rays and a low SNR.[17] The resultant image may have prominent quantum mottle and appear grainy, decreasing the overall image quality (**Fig. 6**).[4,14] The creation, adaptation, and use of technique charts should take the deleterious effects of decreased SNR into

Table 8 Artifacts with lighter areas			
Artifact	**Category**	**Cause**	**Remedy**
Paradoxic overexposure effect	Exposure	Severe overexposure	Reduce exposure technique as needed
Grid cutoff	Exposure	Incorrect grid placement	Correctly place and orient the grid before exposure
Light leak	Postexposure	Imaging plate exposed to visible light	Read images shortly after exposure Avoid manually opening cassettes after exposure

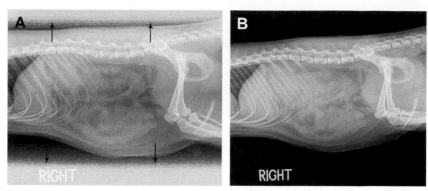

Fig. 4. Right lateral radiographs of an otter, using direct DR. A radiograph was first acquired with the focusing grid oriented upside down (*A*). The lead strips are oriented in a cranial to caudal direction and cause increased attenuation of the divergent x-ray beam ventrally and dorsally (*black arrows*). The radiograph was repeated after correcting grid orientation and does not demonstrate grid cutoff (*B*).

consideration. DR and CR equipment may display a technique factor or value representative of the amount of exposure to the imaging plate or detector.[1] Achieving values within the manufacturer's recommended range is intended to avoid underexposure or overexposure. Image filtering provides a method to alter the conspicuity of quantum mottle. Blurring techniques reduce the prominence of quantum mottle at the expense of decreased image detail. Edge-enhancing techniques increase

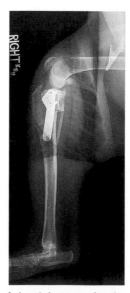

Fig. 5. Mediolateral radiograph of the right crus of a dog and ventrodorsal radiograph of the thorax of a different dog, using CR. The imaging plate was used for 2 different studies without being read or erased in between. There is superimposition of both images. Image processing allows the summated area to be displayed with moderate shades of gray, even though it received double the amount of x-rays.

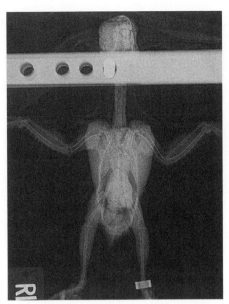

Fig. 6. Ventrodorsal whole-body radiograph of a parrot in a restraining device, using direct DR. Given the patient size, a low exposure technique was used. The entire radiograph is underexposed. It has a diffusely grainy appearance due to quantum mottle artifact.

delineation of object borders as well as underlying quantum mottle.[1,18] Appropriate use of equipment-specific technique charts and prudent use of image filtering techniques are recommended to decrease the quantum mottle artifact.

Saturation

DR and CR have a larger dynamic range when compared with FS. The lower end of the dynamic range is limited by prominence of noise, and the upper end of the dynamic range is limited by saturation.[1,2] Imaging plates and detector arrays record a latent image by storing energy proportional to the amount of x-rays incident per unit area, and there are physical limits to the amount of energy that can be stored. When the maximum storage capacity of an F-center (CR) or detector element (DR) has been reached, the corresponding pixel appears completely black (see **Table 7**).[14] Further increases in x-ray exposure have no effect on areas of saturation.[14] Regions of the patient with less attenuation may appear completely black before processing, and this information is not retrievable by image manipulation or enhancement techniques. Reducing exposure levels is recommended to remain within the dynamic range of the image detector and avoid saturation artifact.

Paradoxic Overexposure Effect

When functioning within the system's dynamic range, areas of a radiograph with larger amounts of exposure appear darker. When using indirect DR, the contrary has been observed in areas of severe overexposure (see **Table 8**).[12] Further increasing the amount of exposure results in a lighter image. This is mostly likely to occur at the edge of thick or dense regions of interest, for which higher exposure techniques are used (**Fig. 7**). The cause for this paradoxic reversal in grayscale relative to exposure has not been determined. When this artifact is recognized, it is often not detrimental

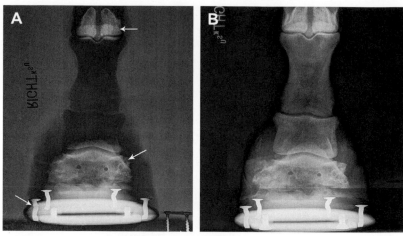

Fig. 7. Dorsopalmar radiograph of the right front foot of a horse, using indirect DR. The initial radiograph was severely overexposed (*A*) and demonstrated paradoxic overexposure effect. Grayscale reversal was present throughout the majority of the radiograph. Only areas of highest x-ray attenuation (*white arrows*) were displayed with normal grayscale. The radiograph was repeated using lower exposure settings (*B*) and had a decreased amount of artifact.

to image interpretation. Using techniques with increased x-ray penetration (higher kVp) and decreased total number of x-rays (lower mAs) may decrease the frequency of paradoxic overexposure effect while maintaining similar overall opacity.

Planking

The digital array of most DR systems is divided into separate sections, each with a separate amplifier. The amplifiers multiply the amount of detected signal to decrease the number of x-rays needed for image formation and, therefore, decrease patient exposure and scatter production. Equipment calibration is performed to regulate these amplifiers and result in a more uniform image.[14] The mild differences in amplification between adjacent sections should not be noticeable when using moderate exposure techniques. Overexposure may allow the calibration mask to become visible and demonstrate differences in the shade of gray between one section and the next (see **Table 6**).[14] The separate sections usually appear as rectangular planks (see **Fig. 1**).[14] Planking artifact has been observed in coincidence with paradoxic overexposure effect.[12] Decreasing the number of incident x-rays (lower mAs) may help avoid planking. Initial calibration and scheduled maintenance are recommended.

Radiofrequency Interference

Detector arrays are constructed with shielding that blocks radiofrequency (RF) interference. RF interference may originate from within the DR system or extraneous sources.[14] Large amounts of RF interference, proximity to the source, and breaks in RF shielding make artifact production more likely (see **Table 6**). RF interference artifacts may occur intermittently, making identification of their cause more difficult.[14] They usually appear as repetitive linear streaks of lighter and darker shades of gray. Distancing the detector array from RF sources and maintaining an intact, functional RF shield will eliminate associated artifacts.

POSTEXPOSURE ARTIFACTS
Light Leak

When using CR, imaging plates are exposed, read, and then erased by visible light. The erasure process liberates energy stored in the imaging plate and removes the latent image. If an imaging plate is exposed to visible light after x-ray exposure but before reading, a fraction of its latent image may be removed (see **Table 8**).[12] Noticeable erasure by ambient light may take several minutes. This is opposite to the effect seen in FS, where subjecting a film to light before developing will lead to severe darkening. If light strikes only a portion of the imaging plate, the uneven and incomplete erasure may be more prominent (**Fig. 8**). If the entire imaging plate is subjected to visible light, the image may appear diffusely underexposed and of poor quality. Light-leak artifacts have been observed when servicing cassettes or imaging plates before the reading process occurs. Light-leak artifacts can be avoided by maintaining functional cassettes and readers and minimizing exposure of imaging plates to light sources.

Fading

A latent image is created using CR by exciting molecules within the imaging plate when exposed to x-rays. The trapped energy of the excited molecules is intended to be released by a red laser during the reading process and result in a proportionate release of green light.[11] If an imaging plate is not read shortly after being exposed, the excited molecules in the imaging plate will gradually lose their energy and return to a neutral state. The latent image will slowly be lost (see **Table 3**).[7] Reading an imaging plate several days after exposure will result in an image that may appear grainy, underexposed, or have generalized decreased quality (**Fig. 9**).[7,11] Newer imaging plates

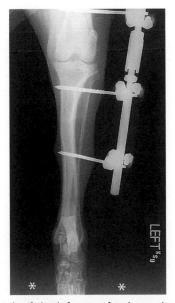

Fig. 8. Craniocaudal radiograph of the left crus of a dog, using CR. A cassette malfunction required servicing in between exposure and reading of the imaging plate. The cassette was partially opened on the side corresponding to the distal aspect of the latent image. Ambient light entered this side of the cassette and caused loss of stored energy. The distal aspect of the radiograph (*) appears lighter.

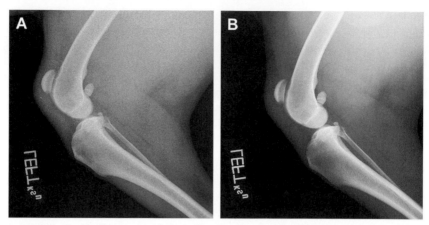

Fig. 9. Mediolateral radiographs of the stifle of a dog, using CR. One of the imaging plates (*A*) was read 7 d after storage in a location free of light and protected from radiation. Fading artifact is present and manifests as a diffusely grainy image of decreased overall quality. The imaging plate read shortly after exposure (*B*) does not exhibit this artifact.

have more stable forms of energy storage and are less susceptible to fading.[7] Fading artifacts can be avoided by immediately reading imaging plates after each exposure.

READING ARTIFACTS
Debris

Radiographs made with CR and FS may exhibit a similar artifact when debris is present in the cassette (see **Table 4**).[4,10] With either system, it appears as a sharply demarcated, white representation of the trapped material (**Fig. 10**).[3,9,10] The debris

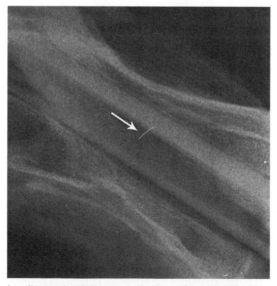

Fig. 10. Right lateral radiograph of the cervical spine of a horse during myelography, using CR. Close-up of the vertebral canal at the level of C2. A hair (*white arrow*) was present on the imaging plate during the reading process and blocked light emission from the imaging plate. It resulted in a linear white artifact.

artifact may mimic foreign material or mineral fragments. With FS, the artifact is due to blockage of light emitted by the intensifying screen during the exposure process. Debris artifacts in CR are usually created during the reading process. Any material on the surface of the imaging plate will block emitted light from reaching the photomultiplier tube, which is used to read the latent image.[9,10] CR cassettes should only be opened during reading or maintenance. Routine cleaning should be performed carefully and in compliance with manufacturer's recommendations.

Dirty Light Guide

During the imaging plate reading process, a red laser strikes the imaging plate one line at a time. The imaging plate releases its stored energy in the form of a green light, and this light is directed through a light guide and into the photomultiplier tube. Blockage of light within the light guide will impede the released energy from reaching the photomultiplier tube along a tract in the direction of imaging plate translation through the reader (see **Table 4**).[3] This will appear as a longitudinal white line over the image **(Fig. 11)**.[9,17] The light guide should be cleaned routinely during scheduled maintenance and as needed to prevent dirty light guide artifacts.[3]

Skipped Scan Lines

The imaging plate is slowly moved through the imaging plate reader while it is struck by a laser and releases its stored energy one line at a time. The imaging plate is moved at a predetermined and reliable rate. Abrupt alterations in the rate of translation may result in incorrect object representation or omission of information.[10] Skipped scan line artifacts usually manifest as the absence of the thin portion of the image and apposition of the remaining image on either side (see **Table 6**). This may appear as foreshortening or step malalignment of an object. It is caused by physical jarring of the

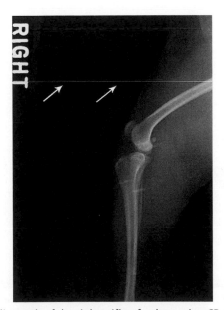

Fig. 11. Mediolateral radiograph of the right stifle of a dog, using CR. Dirt was present on the light guide, blocked transmission of light from the imaging plate to the photomultiplier tube, and resulted in a white line (*white arrows*) along the length of the image.

imaging plate reader or fluctuations in supplied power during the reading process.[4] Stable imaging plate reader mechanics and power supply may reduce the occurrence of this artifact. CR equipment should always be handled carefully.

Moiré

Images made with CR and DR are read and created one line at a time. The number of lines read per unit distance is the sampling frequency and differs between radiographic equipment. Objects of regularly repeated attenuation also have an inherent frequency. The frequency of scatter reduction grids is equal to the number of lead strips per unit distance. When a static grid is imaged, the grid frequency and sampling frequency may intersect in a series of points of higher attenuation and create the impression of straight or curved lines throughout the image (**Fig. 12**) (see **Table 4**).[10,17,19] These white lines may be of a thickness and orientation different from the lead strips in the grid. Coiled metallic objects in patient monitoring or anesthetic equipment can also create this artifact.[10] The distorted grid lines superimposed over the image may obscure the region of interest. Moiré artifact occurs most frequently with stationary grids of low density (lines per inch) that are oriented near parallel to the direction of readout.[2] Malfunction of the grid oscillation or its timing mechanism has led to artifact production. Use of a high-density, oscillating Bucky grid oriented perpendicular to the detector or imaging plate readout direction should decrease production of Moiré artifact.[3,9]

WORKSTATION ARTIFACTS
Faulty Transfer

When using CR and DR, data from imaging plate readers and the detector array are transferred to the workstation. Correct representation of the patient relies on the unadulterated transfer of approximately 4 to 32 MB of data from the image-capturing

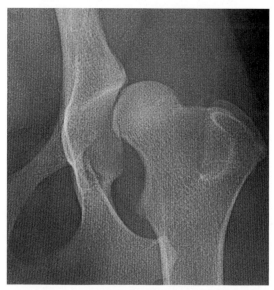

Fig. 12. Ventrodorsal radiograph of the pelvis of a dog, using direct DR. Close-up of the left coxofemoral joint. Curved, thin, white lines are present throughout the image due to grid and sampling frequency interference, moiré artifact.

device to the workstation. Aberrations of information can be due to memory, digitization, or communication errors and result in distortion or misplacement of the region of interest (see **Table 6**).[17] Distortion artifacts alter the appearance of the object and can appear as parallel streaks, elongation, or replacement of portions of the image with areas that are completely black or white (**Fig. 13**).[12] Images with misplacement artifacts are characterized by incorrect localization of fractions of the radiographs throughout the image. Fractions may be duplicated or superimposed over each other.[12] Faulty transfer may be due to fluctuations in power or loose data cables. The instigating cause is often transient, and repeat radiographs may not demonstrate artifact. Wireless communication may result in faulty transfer errors and is discouraged. To avoid artifacts associated with faulty transfer, a reliable method of data transfer, stable connections, and secure power source should be used.

Border Detection

Most DR and CR equipment do not have integrated communication between the x-ray tube head and the detector or imaging plate. The amount of x-ray collimation and desired image size are unknown by the workstation. There are multiple levels of automation that can be performed by the workstation to detect collimation margins and crop the radiograph accordingly. When processing the image, radiograph borders may be applied to the image erroneously, leading to partial omission of the image or inclusion of the area outside the primary x-ray field (see **Table 7**). Incorrect border detection most frequently occurs at the margin of highly attenuating objects and when an imaging plate is rotated more than 3° relative to the collimated field.[4,7,17] Portions of the object excluded from the image are not included in histogram analysis and postprocessing.[14] This may lead to suboptimal alterations in image display (**Fig. 14**).[4,7,10] Using separate sections of the same imaging plate for multiple radiographs is not recommended and may lead to border detection and postprocessing errors.[17] Using semiautomatic border detection is usually recommended to decrease artifact occurrence. When border detection artifact is present, border delineation can be removed, or the image can be reprocessed with deactivated border detection.

Diagnostic Specifier

Digital radiographs can be manipulated after exposure to enhance their appearance, and this is referred to as postprocessing. Initial manipulation of the radiographs is

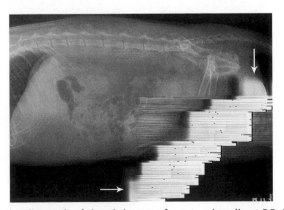

Fig. 13. Right lateral radiograph of the abdomen of a cat, using direct DR. Faulty transfer of information has led to derangement of the bottom right quadrant of the image (*white arrows*). There is distortion of the image and repetitive linear streaks of black and white.

usually computer automated and a product of histogram analysis using specified lookup tables. The histogram is a graphic representation of the amplitude of every opacity throughout the image. Lookup tables are designed to apply image altering techniques, based on the histogram, to display optimal grayscale, contrast, and detail. During equipment setup, different postprocessing techniques are applied depending on the region of interest.[17] Postprocessing usually differs between thoracic, abdominal, and extremity radiographs. When acquiring a radiograph, the area of interest should be designated at the workstation. This will also dictate which postprocessing techniques will be used. Incorrect selection of an area of interest will apply suboptimal postprocessing techniques to the image (see **Table 3**). The overall quality may be decreased and appear as a generalized alteration of opacity, contrast, or detail (**Fig. 15**).[7,10,14] These errors can be easily detected if the selected area of interest is a displayed demographic on the image. Suboptimal postprocessing can also be compensated by manual processing at the viewing station or reprocessing with the correct lookup table at the workstation.[7] Repeating the radiograph is usually not necessary. Selecting the correct area of interest before each radiograph will help in avoiding diagnostic specifier artifacts.

Clipping

Most digital radiographs are large files, which may be cumbersome to transfer, process, and store. Raw data are often 12 to 14 bits.[14] After an image is processed, some of this information is discarded. Information pertinent to accurate patient depiction may be erroneously clipped (see **Table 7**). The final image is often 10 to 12 bits.[14] Clipping usually appears as complete darkening of areas of higher x-ray exposure. Clipping differs from saturation artifact, because it is a product of image processing and occurs within the dynamic range of CR and DR equipment. Processing techniques

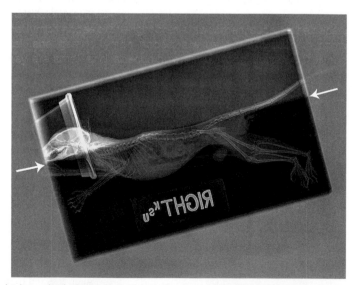

Fig. 14. Right lateral whole-body radiograph of a sugar glider, using CR. The imaging plate and x-ray field of view are not parallel. During processing, the patient's spine was incorrectly identified as an image border (*white arrows*). Border detection artifact presented as inclusion of only the dorsal tissues in the framed image. The remainder of the image ventral to the spine appeared darker and was not included in histogram analysis.

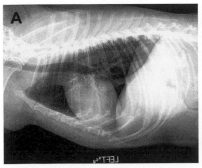 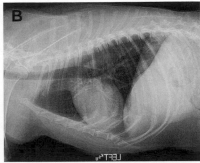

Fig. 15. Left lateral thoracic radiograph of a dog, using direct DR. The radiograph was acquired using the incorrect diagnostic specifier (*A*), which led to processing using parameters chosen for the appendicular skeleton. The image was repeated after selection of the correct region of interest (*B*) and resulted in a radiograph with preferred display for thoracic interpretation.

can be modified at the workstation to include information from these areas. However, manipulation of the image at the display station cannot retrieve information omitted due to clipping artifact.[14] Workstation setup is recommended to customize processing techniques performed for each radiographic study type.

Density Threshold

When objects of extreme density are included in histogram analysis and application of the lookup table, the displayed grayscale is widened to include these objects.[9] This is most likely to affect DR and CR images when metallic implants are present.[7,10] The remaining biologic tissues appear dark and have decreased contrast between them (see **Table 7**). Limits can be placed to exclude objects above a specified density from image analysis. Any object above the density threshold will appear entirely white. Postprocessing will account only for objects below the set threshold, namely biologic tissues, and allow for their improved display. Density thresholds should be implemented to sufficiently exclude extremely dense objects and maintain acceptable contrast in the remainder of the image.

Überschwinger

Improved delineation of object borders increases conspicuity and aids in their identification. Postprocessing techniques that outline the edges of objects can be implemented. This is often beneficial when counterbalancing the decreased contrast that

Table 9 Artifacts with black lines			
Artifact	**Category**	**Cause**	**Remedy**
Moiré	Reading	Interference of grid line and sampling frequency	Use an oscillating grid Use a high-density grid Align the grid perpendicular to the sampling frequency
Überschwinger	Workstation	Inclusion of high-density objects Excessive edge enhancement	Use moderate edge enhancement

may accompany the large latitude of digital radiographs.[17] Different degrees of edge enhancement are usually applied dependent on the region of interest. Unsharp masking is an algorithm often employed with DR and CR. The processed image has a thin black line surrounding objects of higher attenuation when they are adjacent to areas of lower attenuation (**Table 9**).[4,9,10,14,20] Highly attenuating objects, such as metallic implants, may have a dark outline of increased thickness when larger amounts of edge enhancement are implemented.[4,20] The dark zone can be misinterpreted as a region of osteolysis.[16] Unlike osteolysis, überschwinger is of uniform thickness and surrounds all metallic implants on the radiograph.[12] Überschwinger artifact should be recognized when present and can be minimized by using moderate amounts of edge enhancement.

SUMMARY

Increased use of DR and CR in veterinary medicine has led to the increased production of artifacts when using these imaging systems. Artifacts can originate from any stage of image creation and are categorized as such: preexposure, exposure, postexposure, reading, and workstation artifacts.

The increased latitude, increased sensitivity, and physics inherent in digital acquisition make DR and CR substantially different from FS. Artifacts created with these systems also differ from each other and must be addressed accordingly. Digital systems rely on dependable transfer, manipulation, and display of images as well as a stable power supply. Damaged or malfunctioning equipment should be repaired or replaced as needed. Following manufacturer's recommendations on equipment use, care, and preventative maintenance will help improve its longevity and proper function.

REFERENCES

1. American College of Radiology. ACR practice guideline for digital radiography 2007. p. 23–57.
2. Williams MB, Krupinski EA, Strauss KJ, et al. Digital radiography image quality: image acquisition. J Am Coll Radiol 2007;4:371–88.
3. Stearns ED. Computed radiography in perspective. NAVTA Journal 2004;53–8.
4. Solomon SL, Jost RG, Glazer HS, et al. Artifacts in computed radiography. Am J Roentgenol 1991;157:181–5.
5. Tucker DM, Souto M, Barnes GT. Scatter in computed radiography. Radiology 1993;188:271–4.
6. Ramamurthy R, Canning CF, Scheetz JP, et al. Impact of ambient lighting intensity and duration on the signal-to-noise ratio of images from photostimulable phosphor plates processed using DenOptix® and ScanX® systems. Dentomaxillofac Radiol 2004;33:307–11.
7. Volpe JP, Storto ML, Andriole KP, et al. Artifacts in chest radiographs with a third-generation computed radiography system. Am J Roentgenol 1996;166:653–7.
8. Hammerstrom K, Aldrich A, Alves L, et al. Recognition and prevention of computed radiography image artifacts. J Digit Imaging 2006;19:226–39.
9. Cesar LJ, Schueler BA, Zink FE, et al. Artefacts found in computed radiography. Br J Radiol 2001;74:195–202.
10. Oestmann JW, Prokop M, Schaefer CM, et al. Hardware and software artifacts in storage phosphor radiography. Radiographics 1991;11:795–805.

11. Bushberg JT, Seibert JA, Leidholdt EM Jr, et al. The essential physics of medical imaging. 2nd edition. Philadelphia: Lippincott Williams & Wilkins; 2002. p. 145–73, 255–316.
12. Jimenez DA, Armbrust LJ, O'Brien RT, et al. Artifacts in digital radiography. Vet Radiol Ultrasound 2008;49:321–32.
13. Chotas HG, Floyd CE, Ravin CE. Memory artifact related to selenium-based digital radiography systems. Radiology 1997;203:881–3.
14. Drost WT, Reese DJ, Hornoff WJ. Digital radiography artifacts. Vet Radiol Ultrasound 2008;49:S48–56.
15. Padgett R, Kotre CJ. Assessment of the effects of pixel loss on image quality in direct digital radiography. Phys Med Biol 2004;49:977–86.
16. Lo WY, Puchalski SM. Digital imaging processing. Vet Radiol Ultrasound 2008;49: S42–7.
17. Willis CE, Thompson SK, Shepard SJ. Artifacts and misadventures in digital radiography. Appl Radiol 2004;33:11–20.
18. Huda W, Slone RM, Belden CJ, et al. Mottle on computed radiographs of the chest in pediatric patients. Radiology 1996;199:249–52.
19. Lin C, Lee W, Chen S, et al. A study of grid artifacts formation and elimination in computed radiographic images. J Digit Imaging 2006;0:1–11.
20. Tan TH, Boothroyd AE. Uberschwinger artefact in computed radiographs. Correspondence: Br J Radiol 1997;70:431.

PACS and Image Storage

Laura J. Armbrust, DVM

KEYWORDS

- Digital radiography
- Picture archiving and communication system
- Digital imaging • Digital imaging communications in medicine
- Radiology information system

Digital radiography necessitates entirely different methods of image storage, retrieval, and transmission from those of film-screen radiography. This can be confusing and difficult to understand the differing technologies and terminologies. This article focuses on understanding the picture archiving and communication system (PACS), digital imaging communications in medicine (DICOM), radiology information system (RIS)/hospital information system (HIS), and image archiving, retrieval, and transmission.

PICTURE ARCHIVING AND COMMUNICATION SYSTEM

A PACS function is the display, manipulation, archiving, and distribution (communication) of medical digital images.[1–3] Although this may sound like a fairly simple explanation, the implementation is quite complex. The PACS includes both the hardware and software designed for image importation into the system, display, annotation, storage, and communication/transmission functions. The PACS integrates diagnostic images with other related information such as patient demographics, reports, and clinical history.[1,3]

The hardware components include the connection with the image modalities (digital radiographic (DR), computed radiography, CT, ultrasound [US], magnetic resonance imaging [MRI], etc), server, imaging workstations, network lines, and storage devices. The software component has database and workflow management functions as well as image viewing and manipulation capabilities. From the database/workflow management standpoint, the PACS provides for archival, retrieval, and transmission to multiple viewing stations around the hospital via a local area network.[1,3] Connectivity for outside transmission for image interpretation (teleradiology), storage, or web viewing can be performed as well. (**Fig. 1**) One of the greatest benefits of implementing a PACS is that it can provide multiple simultaneous access to images,

Department of Clinical Sciences, Kansas State University, College of Veterinary Medicine, Veterinary Medical Teaching Hospital, 1800 Denison Avenue, Manhattan, KS 66506, USA
E-mail address: armbrust@vet.ksu.edu

Vet Clin Small Anim 39 (2009) 711–718
doi:10.1016/j.cvsm.2009.04.004
0195-5616/09/$ – see front matter © 2009 Elsevier Inc. All rights reserved.

PACS

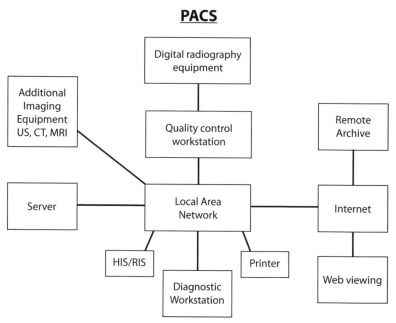

Fig. 1. Schematic of the components of a PACS (picture archive and communication system). Digital imaging equipment produces images that are subsequently managed in a database for image archiving and viewing at multiple locations. A HIS/RIS (hospital and radiology information system) can be integrated to enhance connectivity of the imaging with the hospital management system in a paperless medical record environment.

whereas in the analog (film) world, there is only a single set of films that can be viewed at only one location. A PACS does reduce the staffing time required to manage the film file room, but personnel time is still required to manage the computer system and workflow issues.[1,4]

PACS software vary in image display capabilities and functionality. Image viewing software allows for manipulations of the images on the imaging workstations, with features including zooming, contrast and brightness (window width and window leveling) adjustments, annotations and marking, and measuring functions (**Fig. 2**).

The communication between the PACS and the imaging modalities can be better appreciated if the following parameters are understood: Internet Protocol (IP) address, Application Entity Title (AE title), and assigned communication port. The IP address is unique to each computer and is used for network identification. The AE title is also unique and relates to the program on the computer. The port is the specific computer entry and exit point through which the image information is allowed to travel. TCP/IP (Transmission Control Protocol/Internet Protocol) is another term that may be encountered. TCP/IP is the communication protocol for communication between computers connected to the Internet and is considered the industry standard for network communication.[1,3] These are all parameters that will need to be set up when making the actual connections.[3] Complete network configurations are beyond the scope of this article, but recognize that having a fast network with modern switches will provide rapid image transmission and minimize data transfer errors.

The term mini-PACS is sometimes used for smaller PACS. Mini-PACS are generally designed to handle a smaller number of imaging modalities and image examinations; they have smaller storage capabilities and can be interfaced with a fewer number of

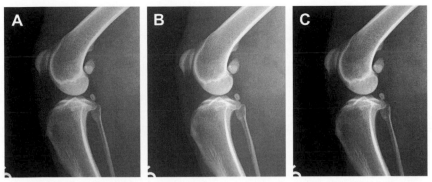

Fig. 2. Image (*A*) is the original image of a stifle. Image (*B*) shows the same stifle after an adjustment in window level (to increase the brightness). In image (*C*) the window width (contrast) has been increased. These functions in image viewing are one of the major benefits of digital imaging systems and come as standard software in PACS.

workstations. Mini-PACS often do not have the same degree of connectivity with other network systems as a fully functioning PACS. The mini-PACS will generally have the same basic viewing functions. There are significant costs associated with purchasing and maintaining a PACS. If a smaller PACS version is purchased, it is wise to determine if it can be easily expanded in the future. In general, PACS upgrades and maintenance can be costly and should be a major consideration when purchasing digital imaging equipment.

DIGITAL IMAGING COMMUNICATIONS IN MEDICINE

DICOM is a specific image file format, analogous to the joint photographic experts group (JPEG) format and tagged image file format commonly used in manipulation and storage of digital camera images. DICOM was conceived in the early 1980s to provide interconnectivity between medical imaging devices from various vendors (CT, MRI, ultrasound, nuclear medicine, and digital radiography) and the multiple viewing and archiving systems. The National Electrical Manufacturers Association (NEMA) and the American College of Radiology were responsible for the inception of DICOM after realizing the need for compatibility between imaging equipment and software.[5,6] This interconnectivity requires that a standard format is used for all medical images. In other words, the cassette-based digital radiography system from vendor A and the cassetteless digital radiography system from vendor B should be viewable using software from vendor C.

In 1993 DICOM 3.0 was released, and since then, it has had many supplements and changes, almost on a monthly basis, to address new technology.[5] It is now considered the international standard in human medicine, and all imaging vendors should adhere to this format.[5] There is currently no requirement for DICOM conformance in veterinary medicine, but it is strongly recommended that all systems should provide a DICOM conformance statement.[6]

The conformance statements can be very lengthy and difficult to evaluate. For a better understanding of DICOM, consider the following terms: DICOM objects and DICOM service class. The DICOM object is essentially the image. DICOM service classes have different roles and can be divided into service class users and service class providers.[5,6] In certain instances, such as sending an image from the imaging modality to the PACS server, the digital radiography machine is the user and the PACS server the provider. In another example, if you are at an imaging workstation and query for archived images, the workstation is the user and the storage server is the provider, but once the image is actually sending, the roles reverse so that the server is the user and the workstation the provider.

The reason to understand the service class providers is that not all systems have the same capabilities. The main DICOM service class options for veterinary medicine include storage, print, and query/retrieve options. Additional options include modality worklist and grayscale display function.[1,3,6] The modality worklist option allows for communication between the HIS or RIS and the image modality. A HIS or RIS allows the patient information to automatically populate the data entry page of the image modality as the study is being set up. This decreases the errors that occur when manually typing in the patient information at multiple locations.[6] The grayscale display function allows for calibration of the viewing monitors at regular intervals. Because many veterinary hospitals are switching to paperless medical record systems, the modality worklist will become more important with time.

Vendors stating that they are DICOM conformant is almost meaningless. Identifying specifically which of the service class options listed above will be provided is of utmost importance to truly understanding the final product.[3,6,7] This information should be available in the vendor DICOM conformance statement.

In addition to standardizing connectivity, the DICOM format provides important security features to help ensure that the images are authentic. To ensure appropriate security, each image must have its own unique identifying number. Any changes to the images can be tracked, which is a necessity when dealing with images as part of the patient's medical record. Complete and up to date information on DICOM can be found on the NEMA Web site.[8]

HOSPITAL INFORMATION SYSTEM AND RADIOLOGY INFORMATION SYSTEM

In an ideally paperless medical record system, the medical record and images are linked. A HIS or RIS allows for this connection.[3] Patient information can be viewed at the PACS image workstations. Conversely, the digital images can be linked with each patient's electronic file. The patient demographics would only need to be entered once, and this information could be communicated to various workstations to avoid multiple manual inputs, thus decreasing the potential for errors in patient data. In human medicine, the data error rate is roughly 20% to 30%, which could result in critical errors and, theoretically, loss of patient information.[1] If a modality worklist can be generated at a digital imaging workstation by communicating with a HIS/RIS, then error rates are decreased as is the time required to enter data or correct mistakes.

Although this connectivity is not commonly used in veterinary practice, it is becoming increasingly used. Just as DICOM 3 format is the image file standard, there is a standard used in human medicine for transfer of text communication between systems. This standard for text is termed Health Language 7.[1,3,7] RIS systems that allow for web-based viewing are helpful if teleradiology is used so that patient information can be viewed by the radiologist. The RIS/HIS ideally allow for storage of many different file types so that in addition to radiographic images, video clips (such as lameness and neurologic examinations or ultrasound clips), endoscopic and laparoscopic images, ECG tracings, and audio files could also be linked to the patient record.[3]

DATA TRANSMISSION, ARCHIVING, AND RETRIEVAL

Efficient communication between modalities, the PACS server, and the Internet all require up to date, high-speed network connections. The network bandwidth is often the greatest bottleneck that inhibits workflow.[9] Hiring an information technology consultant is recommended for initial installation. Investing in high-speed, commercial grade switches, routers, and cable can save time and prevent the frustration of having all new equipment that is slow or virtually nonfunctional. If Internet connectivity is used, it is important for security purposes to have both hardware and software firewalls. Further information on network connections is available.[9]

Once the digital images are acquired and viewed at the quality control workstation (at the digital radiography modality), they are transferred to a server. The server's function is to catalog the images in a database for easy retrieval. Most of these systems allow for various queries: patient name, patient identification, study date, modality, and body part.[3] Images are transmitted to the interpretation workstation for review. Some servers can also be connected to the Internet, allowing viewing via a Web browser at multiple outside locations.

Data compression is generally used to decrease file size to speed transmission and increase storage capacity. File sizes for a two-view radiographic study can easily be 16 MB, which will result in slow transmission times and require large amounts of storage space. Data compression methods include reversible (lossless) and irreversible (lossy) techniques. In both situations, the method used should not result in reduction in diagnostic quality.[3,10–15] A compression ratio can be used to describe the degree of compression based on file size.[11,14] For example, if a 20-MB image is compressed 4:1, the compressed image file size is 5 MB. Lossless compression is limited to a compression ratio of approximately 5:1, while lossy techniques can be up to 100:1.[11] Compression ratios of 10:1 or up to 20:1 usually do not sacrifice image quality; however, an exact compression ratio cannot be given, as there will be variation between images.[11,14,15] It is recommended that images be reviewed on a regular basis to ensure that clinical image quality is maintained.[10,13] Standard JPEG compression can be used for client viewing but should not be used for image interpretation services such as teleradiology. A different form of lossy compression, JPEG 2000, uses wavelet techniques that provide excellent quality at high compression ratios. This method is considered the standard for lossy compression and is commonly used for storage.[11,14] JPEG-LS is a standard form of lossless compression.[14] Whatever form of compression is used, the images should be in a file format that can be transferred to another system if vendor software changes over time.

The PACS should have an appropriate amount of storage space and comply with state regulations regarding medical record retention. Storage may be on-site or off-site. Either way, there should be redundancy in the system so that the data are not lost if there is system failure or damage to the facility. Most modern servers will have hardware redundancy for array controllers, hard drives, and power supply. There are many storage options for both on- and off-site redundancy, including magnetic tape, spinning disks (hard drive, zip drive), optical media (digital versatile disk [DVD], compact disk [CD], Blu-ray), or solid state (universal serial bus [USB] or flash cards).[3,16] Redundant array of independent disk (RAID) servers create an internal backup that provides protection against equipment failure. These can be expensive to purchase and maintain. DVD/CDs are inexpensive, but backing up studies is time consuming and, therefore, may not get done on a daily basis. In addition, it becomes a challenge to manually find cases on DVD/CDs depending on your filing system. External hard drives and USB storage devices have greater storage capabilities but have the same limitations as CD/DVDs. Off-site storage is often an easier option. Costs for off-site storage include the initial setup, high-speed Internet connections, and the ongoing cost of the service. If the company goes out of business, then image data must be retrieved and redistributed; therefore, you should make sure the data are stored in a vendor-independent format. The other big consideration is whether the storage will be on-line or off-line. The term on-line storage is used if the data are readily accessible for viewing. Off-line storage requires that the archived images be restored to an on-line status before viewing, thereby requiring a longer time period for retrieval. Choosing the appropriate method for storage can be difficult, because there are so many options that vary in storage capacity and cost. (**Table 1**) No matter what method is chosen, it should be easily amenable to expansion, as it is common to initially underestimate storage requirements. More in-depth information on storage of digital images is available.[16]

The data file for each image should include the patient data, record number, accession number, examination date, type of examination, and the clinic name. It is important that prior images are retrievable from the archives for a time period appropriate for the clinical needs of a particular patient. Network and software security protocols to protect patient confidentiality and appropriate user accessibility and authentication must be met.[3,9] Patient data entry is never 100% correct, so server software should allow for editing certain tags in the image headers. For security purposes, this should be reserved only for specified authorized personnel. DICOM protocol requires the editing be documented so that it can be traced over time.[3,10]

DIGITAL IMAGE VIEWING

Digital images can be viewed in house, or the systems have the ability to create a CD that contains the DICOM files embedded in a DICOM image viewer, which can be viewed with a traditional personal computer at other locations. These CDs can then be distributed to clients or used for referral and teleradiology purposes.[3] Another method of viewing is via a web-based browser. These browsers are not generally used for image interpretation but for viewing images with clients or in examination rooms and surgical suites. In this case, the images are usually compressed, so they have a decreased image quality as described earlier.

Table 1				
Archiving methods used for digital imaging				
	RAID Server	**CD/DVD**	**External Hard Drive or USB**	**Off-Site Storage**
Internal vs external backup	Internal	External	External	External
Expense	High	Low	Low	Moderate to high
Maintenance of equipment	High	Low	Low	Low
Daily manual input required	No	Yes	No/yes	No
Access to prior studies	Easy	Difficult	Moderate	Easy
Space	Moderate	Low	Moderate	None
Maintains DICOM integrity	Yes	Yes	Yes	Sometimes (vendor specific)

Redundant array of independent disks provide for internal redundancy. Off-site storage refers to a company storing the images. CD/DVDs and hard drives or USBs can be stored either at the clinic or at an off-site location.

Many teleradiology services are available to veterinarians. The vendors selling the equipment will often provide teleradiology options. As long as the systems have standard DICOM format, various teleradiology services can be used over time. Sending DICOM images via e-mail is not practical due to the large file sizes (10-12 MB/image). Further information on veterinary teleradiology is available.[15]

SUMMARY

A PACS provides a mechanism for digital image management (viewing, transmission, archiving, and retrieval). Image files that are transferred into a PACS are in a DICOM file format, which is the standard in medical imaging. A hospital information system or radiology information system allows for connectivity between an electronic medical system and digital imaging modalities. When switching to an all-digital domain, it is important to consider data security, archiving capabilities, and redundancy of the system with disaster recovery plans.

When purchasing PACS, consider the following questions:

1. DICOM conformance statement:
   a. What is available with the system?
   b. What are the storage, printing, query/retrieve options?
   c. Does the system have a modality worklist and grayscale display function options?
2. Network connections:
   a. Is the system locally limited (intranet) or does it have web-based options (Internet)?
   b. Are upgrades available and if so what are their cost and limits of expandability?
   c. Does the system have firewalls and other security devices?
   d. Is there an option for off-site storage or teleradiology?
   e. What type of broadband Internet connection is needed?
   f. What is the minimum upload speed needed (usually Internet connections are described in terms of both download and upload speeds)?
   g. Can the PACS send the images in the background without tying up the workstation for other uses such as viewing?
3. Functionality of the PACS viewing:
   a. What viewing options are available beyond the standard brightness, contrast, zoom, pan, measurements, and so forth?
4. Data redundancy:
   a. What is the method of on-site and off-site storage and what are the associated costs?
   b. Is off-site storage on-line or off-line?
   c. How quickly can archived images be viewed?
   d. What type of image compression is used?
5. What are the requirements for long-term medical record storage in your state?
6. Options for burning CD/DVD
   a. Is there a method of burning CD/DVDs for storage or distribution to clients?
   b. Is an auto-opening viewer included in the final CDs?
7. Teleradiography
   a. Are teleradiology services available via the vendor?
   b. Can images be sent in a format that is viewable by any teleradiology service?
   c. Can the system easily autoroute images without downtime?

REFERENCES

1. Oosterwijk H. PACS fundamentals. Aubrey (TX): Otech Inc.; 2004. p. 11–20.
2. Bansal GJ. Digital radiography. A comparison with modern conventional imaging. Postgrad Med J 2006;82:425–8.
3. Robertson ID, Saveraid T. Hospital, radiology, and picture archiving and communication systems. Vet Radiol Ultrasound 2008;49(1 Supp 1):S19–28.
4. Siegel E, Reiner B. Computers in radiology-Workflow redesign: the key to success when using PACS. AJR Am J Roentgenol 2002;178:563–6.
5. Oosterwijk H, Gihring PT. DICOM basics. 3rd edition. Aubrey (TX): Otech Inc.; 2005. p. 9–18.
6. Wright MA, Balance D, Robertson ID, et al. Introduction to DICOM for the practicing veterinarian. Vet Radiol Ultrasound 2008;49(1 Supp 1):S14–8.
7. Digital x-ray systems, Part 1: an introduction to DX technologies and an evaluation of cassette DX systems. Health Devices 2001;30(8):273–84.
8. Available at: http://www.nema.org/stds/ps3set.cfm. Accessed September 8, 2008.
9. Ballance D. The network and its role in digital imaging and communications in medicine imaging. Vet Radiol Ultrasound 2008;49(1 Supp 1):S29–32.
10. American College of Radiology. Practice guideline for digital radiography. Reston (VA): American College of Radiology; 2007. p. 23–57.
11. Seeram E. Digital image compression. Radiol Technol 2005;76(6):449–59.
12. American College of Radiology. ACR technical standard for digital image data management. Reston (VA): American College of Radiology; 2002. p. 811–9.
13. American College of Radiology. ACR technical standard for teleradiology. Reston (VA): American College of Radiology; 2005. p. 801–10.
14. Koff DA, Shulman H. An overview of digital compression of medical images: can we use lossy image compression in radiology? Can Assoc Radiol J 2006; 57(4):211–7.
15. Poteet BA. Veterinary teleradiology. Vet Radiol Ultrasound 2008;49(1 Supp 1): S33–6.
16. Wallack S. Digital image storage. Vet Radiol Ultrasound 2008;49(1 Supp 1): S37–41.

Nontraditional Interpretation of Lung Patterns

Peter V. Scrivani, DVM

KEYWORDS

- Lung • Radiography • Computed tomography
- Atelectasis • Dog • Cat

In the 1970s and 1980s, a series of case reports, review articles, and text books established what may be considered as the traditional approach to radiographic interpretation of lung disease in veterinary medicine.[1–16] In the past decade, our group has proposed a modified approach that is referred to as an alternate appraisal or a nontraditional approach.[17–19] It is a work in progress, and we keep modifying the basic premise as new information is gathered. The fundamentals of either approach are very similar, but the major difference is where the emphasis is placed. For example, our group emphasizes that, in most patients, the three most important radiographic signs for prioritizing the differential diagnosis are the opacity of the lung, the degree of lung expansion, and the macroscopic distribution of lung lesions. Additional signs (including the more traditionally emphasized ones), however, are extremely important and still used to prioritize the differential diagnosis. Another difference between the two approaches is that we try to incorporate terminology that reflects current usage in human medicine, which has advanced at a more substantial pace than veterinary medicine—especially with the extensive use of thoracic computed tomography and histopathologic correlation that has aided radiographic interpretation.[20]

To simplify the description for this article, discussion of pulmonary blood-vessel alterations are relegated to the cardiovascular system and therefore discussed only minimally. Additionally, since it is well known that improperly exposed radiographs or unacceptably positioned patients may unfavorably affect radiographic interpretation, assumptions are made that abnormalities detected on thoracic radiographs are localized to the lung (not merely superimposed) and neither due to technical complications nor age-related changes. Herein, describing a lung lesion also implies that the viewer thinks that lung pathology is present. This approach to the radiographic description is reasonable when the radiologic study is considered as if it were

Department of Clinical Sciences, C2512 Veterinary Medical Center, Box 36, College of Veterinary Medicine, Cornell University, Ithaca, NY 14853, USA
E-mail address: pvs2@cornell.edu

Vet Clin Small Anim 39 (2009) 719–732
doi:10.1016/j.cvsm.2009.04.005

a scientific test.[21] If, for example, we assume a "null hypothesis" and anticipate that the radiographic findings will fall within the expected range of normal for the given population, then it is necessary to describe only those findings that are abnormal and disprove the null hypothesis—these findings are referred to as positive findings.[21] The exception occurs when a clinical question implies the possible presence of a specific abnormality and introduces a positive hypothesis that the findings will document the questioned abnormality.[21] In this case, normal findings that refute the presence of the questioned abnormality should be described and are referred to as pertinent negatives.[21]

OPACITY OF THE LUNG AND DEGREE OF LUNG EXPANSION

Altered opacity of the lungs is one of the most common radiographic signs associated with pulmonary disease. Therefore, detecting altered opacity is frequently the first positive finding that the lungs are abnormal. The altered opacity may be either increased (more opaque) or decreased (more lucent), but the majority of pulmonary diseases in dogs and cats produce an increased opacity. Negative findings are possible, because some diseases may produce no alteration of opacity due to the pathogenesis of that particular disease, disease severity, or stage of the disease. In addition, whereas detecting altered opacity of the lung is a sensitive test for lung disease, it is often not specific for the type of lung disease. Therefore, this finding is generally combined with other signs to form a pattern of the disease. One of the most important signs to help further classify the pattern of lung disease is the size of the lungs or lobes, which may be decreased, normal, or increased. Lungs that have decreased size are described as incompletely expanded. Lungs that have normal or increased size are fully expanded.

An incompletely expanded lung that has an increased opacity that completely or partially obscures the margins of pulmonary blood vessels and airway walls is called *collapse* or *atelectasis*. Atelectasis is reduced inflation of all or part of the lung. It is important to differentiate an abnormally opaque lung lobe that is incompletely expanded from one that is fully expanded lung, because this latter pattern always implies pulmonary disease and atelectasis implies either disease or a technical complication that is incidental or may obscure a real lesion. The radiographic signs that alert the viewer to reduced lung volume are a mediastinal shift toward the abnormal appearing lung, crowding and reorientation of pulmonary blood vessels, crowding of ribs, compensatory hyperinflation of other lung lobes, bronchial rearrangement, cardiac rotation, displacement of interlobar fissures, displacement of the diaphragm, change in location of abnormal structures, and rounded pulmonary margins. Not all need to be present to recognize atelectasis (**Fig. 1**).

In some patients, atelectasis may be the most important indicator of disease and not just a technical complication to be dismissed without further consideration. Additionally, if it is just a technical complication associated with prolonged recumbency, anesthesia (**Fig. 2**), or not taking a deep breath, it may be severe enough to obscure an important lesion. There are several types of atelectasis: relaxing, obstructive, adhesive, and cicatrizing.[22] The different types relate to the mechanism for which the lungs cannot inflate. Relaxation atelectasis is due to the unopposed tendency of the lung to collapse due to inherent elasticity. Diseases that may produce this type of atelectasis are pneumothorax, pleural fluid, space-occupying lesion, and gravity-dependent and shallow breathing.[22] Obstructive atelectasis is due to absorption of alveolar gas without replacement due to airway obstruction. The differential diagnosis includes neoplasm (**Fig. 3**), foreign body, mucous plugging (eg, asthma), infectious

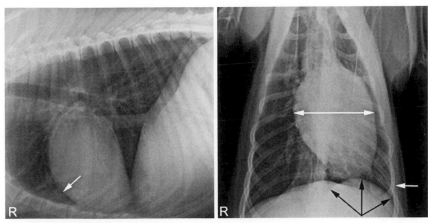

Fig. 1. Orthogonal thoracic radiographs of a 9-year-old, neutered, male Weimaraner with atelectasis. On the lateral view, note the increased opacity that obscures the margins on pulmonary blood vessels (*white arrow*). On the ventrodorsal view, note the mediastinal shift of the heart to the left (*double-headed white arrow*), rib crowding (*white arrow*), and cranial displacement of the left crus of the diaphragm (*black arrows*).

bronchitis or pneumonia (**Fig. 4**), or ciliary diskinesis.[22] Whereas pneumonia typically produces lung consolidation, atelectasis may occur when the lung lobe is not completely filled with pus and exudates obstruct some of the airways, preventing refilling of alveolar gas. Adhesive atelectasis is due to lumen surfaces of alveoli sticking together due to surfactant abnormality. Diseases include neonatal respiratory distress syndrome, acute respiratory distress syndrome, and pulmonary thrombosis.[22] Cicatrizing atelectasis occurs when the lungs do not increase in volume under normal

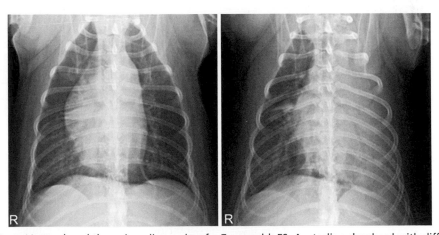

Fig. 2. Ventrodorsal thoracic radiographs of a 7-year-old, FS, Australian shepherd with difficulty breathing due to a pharyngeal mass. The radiograph on the left was obtained while the patient was awake. The radiograph on the right was obtained a day later while the patient was under general anesthesia. Note that, during general anesthesia, the rib cage is not as well expanded, there is a mediastinal shift to the left, and the left lung is small and increased in opacity. The results of that study are indeterminate for lung disease—atelectasis may be due to primary lung disease, secondary to some other disease, or may be a technical complication that is incidental or may obscure a real lesion.

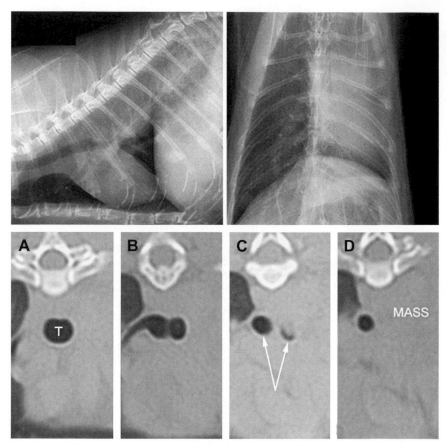

Fig. 3. Orthogonal thoracic radiographs (*top row*) and sequential thoracic CT scans (*bottom row*) of an 11-year-old, neutered, male, domestic longhair cat with left-lung atelectasis due to tumor. The left lung is severely small, causing a mediastinal shift of the heart to the left; the remaining lung is hyperinflated. In this case, atelectasis is due to a mass growing into the left-principal bronchus. On the CT scans, note the two principal bronchi (*arrows*) that are caudal to the tracheal (T) bifurcation. The lung mass extends into and completely obscures the lumen of the left bronchus (the right bronchus remains air filled). The four CT scans are obtained in sequential order from cranial to caudal (*A–D*).

respiration because of reduced compliance due to such things as chronic idiopathic fibrosis, chronic immune-mediated lung disease, chronic pneumonia, and radiation pneumonitis.[22]

It may not be possible to differentiate between the different types of atelectasis simply by observing certain radiographic signs. The cause of atelectasis, however, may be prioritized by noting if the atelectasis is distributed regionally or diffusely. A regional lesion might suggest a local problem such as a foreign body, radiation pneumonitis, or recumbency.[19] A diffuse distribution might suggest diseases that produce cicatrizing atelectasis or incomplete inhalation.[19] Further characterization of atelectasis is probably possible only when the underlying pathogenesis can be determined.

Whereas an incompletely expanded lung lobe may or may not be due to disease, a fully expanded lung that has altered opacity is abnormal and indicates pulmonary disease. If enlarged, the lung lobe may have a convex surface, a rounded contour,

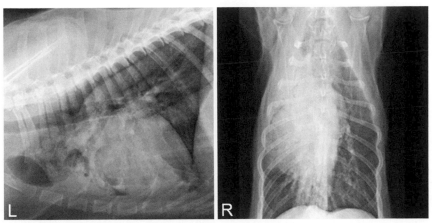

Fig. 4. Orthogonal thoracic radiographs of an 11-year-old, FS, Akita with vomiting, fever, and difficulty breathing attributed to pneumonia. Note that the right-cranial and right-middle lung lobes have an increased opacity that completely obscures pulmonary blood vessels and creates air bronchograms. Additionally, these lung lobes are not fully inflated, as the heart is shifted to the right, and the left-cranial lung lobe is hyperinflated, crossing midline more than normal. In this case, the atelectasis is attributed to aspiration pneumonia.

or displace structures away from it. A fully expanded lung that has a homogeneous increased opacity that obscures the margins of pulmonary blood vessels and airway walls is called *consolidation*: air bronchograms may or may not be present (**Fig. 5**).[20] Consolidation is not an end-point diagnosis but rather refers to a condition where an exudate or other product of disease replaces alveolar air, rendering the lung solid.[20] A fully expanded lung that has a hazy increased opacity that only partially obscures the margins of pulmonary blood vessels and airway walls is called *ground-glass opacity*.[20] This finding is caused by partial filling of air spaces, interstitial thickening (due to fluid,

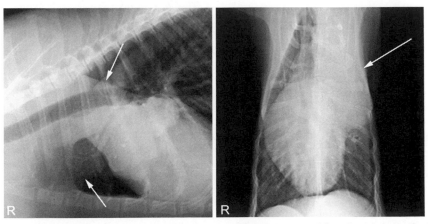

Fig. 5. Orthogonal thoracic radiographs of a 10-year-old, neutered female greyhound with a consolidated cranial part of the left-cranial lung lobe (*arrows*). Note that the abnormal lung lobe is fully expanded and enlarged, displacing the heart away from the abnormal lung lobe (to the *right*).

cells, or fibrosis), increased capillary blood volume, or a combination of these, the common factor being displacement of air.[20] The differential diagnosis for increased opacity in a fully expanded lung includes such diseases as pneumonia, neoplasia, hemorrhage, pulmonary edema, and immune-mediated diseases (**Fig. 6**).

A fully expanded lung that has a decreased opacity (**Fig. 7**) may be due to retention of air in the lung downstream to the obstruction (ie, *air trapping*), reduced pulmonary blood volume (ie, *oligemia* or *hypoperfusion*), or permanently enlarged air spaces downstream to the terminal bronchiole with destruction of the alveolar walls (ie, *emphysema*).[20] Compensatory hyperinflation following collapse or removal of a lung lobe may also appear in this manner.

MACROSCOPIC DISTRIBUTION OF LUNG LESION

The next radiographic sign to incorporate for defining a pattern of lung disease is the macroscopic distribution of the lesion. We emphasize this sign as important, because it is extremely helpful for generating a prioritized differential diagnosis list, easier to teach and learn, and correlates well with gross pathology. Additionally, in people, several lung diseases have been classified using histologic criteria, but the macroscopic distribution of the lesion during computed tomography (CT) is distinct and linked to a specific clinical syndrome.[23] We currently use the following descriptions of macroscopic distribution of lung lesions: cranioventral, caudodorsal, diffuse, lobar, focal, locally extensive, multifocal, and asymmetric. With increasing use of CT, other distributions may be important (eg, central versus peripheral within a lung lobe).

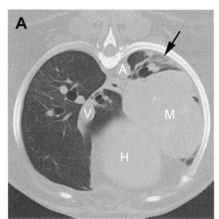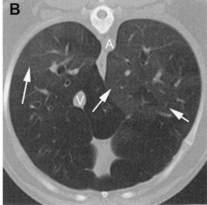

Fig. 6. Thoracic CT Scans of a 14-year-old, neutered female Cocker spaniel (*A*) and a 3-year-old, neutered female West Highland terrier (*B*). In A, note the atelectasis in the left-caudal lung lobe (*black arrow*)—this lung lobe is incompletely inflated and has an increased opacity that partially to completely obscures pulmonary blood vessels. Immediately ventral to this lung lobe there is a lung mass (M). In this situation, the abnormal lung is consolidated, because it is fully inflated, and the increased opacity completely obscures the bronchovascular margins. When atelectasis and consolidation occur concurrently within the lungs, it may be problematic, especially during radiography, to differentiate the conditions. In B, the left- and right-caudal lung lobes have ground-glass opacity, (*arrows*) because the lungs are fully inflated, and bronchovascular margins are only partially obscured. The aorta (A) and caudal vena cava (V) are identified.

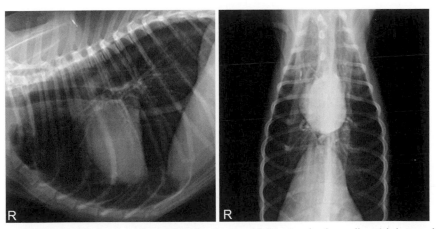

Fig. 7. Orthogonal thoracic radiographs of a 5-year-old, FS, standard poodle with hypovolemia. Note that the lungs are fully expanded and reduced in opacity due to small pulmonary blood vessels.

The cranioventral distribution generally conforms to the region of the left-cranial, right-cranial, and right-middle lung lobes (**Fig. 8**). Not all parts of this region need to be affected to determine that a cranioventral distribution is present. This designation tends to imply that gravity has an effect on the distribution of the lesion, although that is not necessary. If the disease is severe, then a lesion may extend into the ventral part of caudal lung lobes. It is important to note that on the lateral view, the cranioventral lung field actually extends into the caudoventral portion of the thorax and is superimposed on the heart. The caudodorsal distribution generally conforms to the region of the left-caudal, right-caudal, and accessory lung lobes. When severe, this distribution tends toward being diffuse. A *diffuse* distribution implies that all parts of all lung lobes are abnormal (**Fig. 9**). These distributions tend to imply that the lesion is distributed by a hematogenous route or by the airways. On the ventrodorsal view, the cranioventral

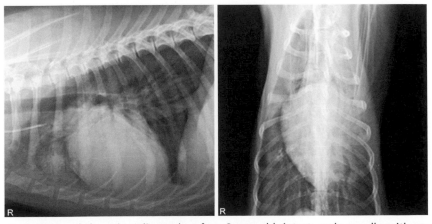

Fig. 8. Orthogonal thoracic radiographs of an 8-year-old, intact, male poodle with pneumonia. Note the cranioventral distribution of the increased opacity, which is worse on the left.

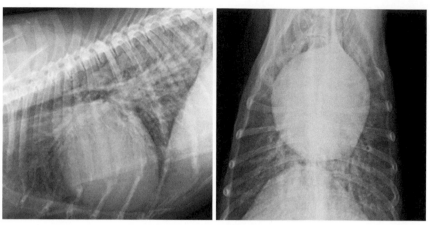

Fig. 9. Orthogonal thoracic radiographs of a 9-year-old, neutered, male, mixed-breed dog with left-sided, congestive heart failure. Note that the increased opacity is distributed in all parts of the lungs but worse caudodorsally (caudodorsal-to-diffuse).

and caudodorsal lung fields overlap at the level of the heart, and it may not be possible to differentiate where the lesion is located without the orthogonal view.

If the lesion is discretely localized to an entire lung lobe, then the term *lobar* may be used (see **Fig. 5**). The term *focal* is used to describe a single lesion that is usually is well defined and discrete and tends to imply diseases like a neoplasm, abscess, granuloma, cyst, hematoma, cavity, bleb, or bulla. If the focus is more of a poorly defined patch, then the term *locally extensive* may be used. The margins may be poorly defined if the adjacent lung is collapsed or if the lesion is more infiltrative. The term *multifocal* is used when there is more than one lesion in one, multiple, or all lung lobes (**Fig. 10**). If all lung lobes are involved, the term multifocal is used when there is some normal lung between lesions (ie, the distribution is not diffuse). These lesions are usually discrete but, alternatively, may be poorly defined patches that have a random distribution.

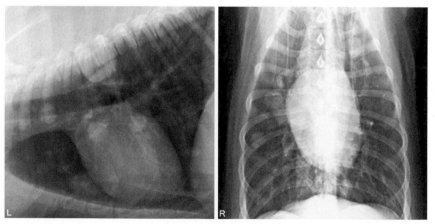

Fig. 10. Orthogonal thoracic radiographs of a 6-year-old, neutered, male Bernese mountain dog with pulmonary metastasis of a prostatic transitional cell carcinoma. In the lungs, there are multiple, well-defined, soft-tissue nodules with a multifocal distribution.

The term *asymmetric* is used to describe lesion distributions that do not conform to one of the other categories (**Fig. 11**). With this designation, there may be one or more lesions that are usually patchy, locally extensive, and poorly defined (but not necessarily); often there is left-right asymmetry. This distribution tends to imply diseases that may occur at random locations within the lungs (eg, cancer, trauma, inflammatory).

APPEARANCES OF INCREASED OPACITY WITHIN THE LUNG

The traditional lung patterns applied to disseminated pulmonary diseases initially were believed to signify in part the microscopic distribution of lesions within the alveoli, interstitium, or bronchi.[1] This idea of describing diffuse pulmonary disease based on histologic classifications, however, is no longer considered reliable or accurate in human medicine, which is one of the reasons we prefer using more wide-ranging terminology.[24–25]

The *interstitium* consists of a continuum of connective tissue throughout the lung, comprising three subdivisions: (1) the bronchovascular interstitium, surrounding and supporting the bronchi, arteries, and veins from the hilum to the level of the respiratory bronchiole; (2) the parenchymal interstitium, situated between alveolar and capillary basement membranes; and (3) the subpleural connective tissue.[20] In people, but not in dogs and cats, the interstitium distinctly also extends into interlobular septa, which may create distinctive lines when abnormal. Since the alveoli and parenchymal interstitium are superimposed on each other in the radiograph, increased thickness of the interstitium, partial filling of the alveoli with fluid or cells, or partial collapse of the alveoli will result in the same amount of attenuation of the x-ray beam. Therefore, simply detecting an increased opacity in the lung does not correlate to a specific microscopic anatomic location. Therefore, more generic terms such as ground-glass opacity and consolidation are preferable, because they do not specify a microscopic anatomic location. Furthermore, many diseases affect multiple microscopic distributions at the same time.

Likewise, the airway wall and bronchovascular interstitium attenuate the x-ray beam as a unit that forms a silhouette on the radiograph; therefore, if the unit is thick, one

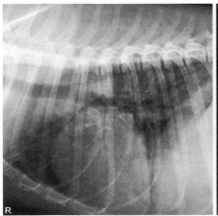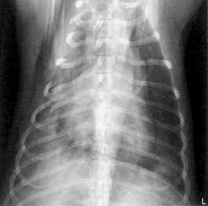

Fig. 11. Orthogonal thoracic radiographs of a 2.5-year-old, neutered, female Jack Russell terrier with pulmonary contusions (hemorrhage) and rib fractures. The distribution of the lung lesions does not conform to any of the described distributions, as it is located in the entire right lung (both cranially and caudally) and focally in the left-caudal-lung lobe.

cannot differentiate a thick airway from thick bronchovascular interstitium. Therefore, the term *bronchocentric* is preferred, as it applies to diseases that are conspicuously centered on macroscopic bronchovascular bundles but does not differentiate between microscopic structures (**Fig. 12**). Previously, we used the term "airway" to describe this radiographic appearance.[18] An increased opacity within the lungs that has a bronchocentric location may be differentiated from increased opacity within the air space, because they have a different appearance. The *air space* is the gas-containing part of the lung, including the respiratory bronchioles but excluding purely conducting airways such as terminal bronchioles. (Bronchioles are non–cartilage-containing airways.)[20] This term is used in conjunction with consolidation, ground-glass opacity, nodules, and masses. Note that there are strong similarities between the radiographic appearances of alveolar, interstitial, and bronchial patterns and consolidation, ground-glass, and bronchocentric opacities. The difference in terminology, however, better suits current understanding of the pathogenesis of these radiographic appearances.

Focal, approximately spherical, discrete lesions may be further characterized by their opacity and size. A *bleb* is a small gas-containing space that is not larger than 1 cm in diameter and located within the visceral pleura or in the subpleural lung.[20] A *bulla* is an air space that is more than 1 cm in diameter, sharply demarcated by a thin wall.[20] A *cavity* is a gas-containing space of unspecified size within pulmonary consolidation, a mass, or a nodule that is usually produced by expulsion or drainage of a necrotic part of the lesion via the bronchial tree (**Fig. 13**).[20] A *nodule* is a rounded, soft-tissue opacity, well or poorly defined, that is up to 3 cm in diameter.[18,20] A tiny nodule (not larger than 3 mm) may be described as a micronodule (or miliary when profuse).[20] A *mass* is any lesion that is larger than 3 cm in diameter without regard to contour, border, or density characteristics.[18,20] Note that these size recommendations are made for humans, and clinical judgment should be exercised when applying these criteria to dogs and cats that have variable body sizes. Nevertheless, it is useful to know that the differentiation between these descriptions is often based on differences in size and opacity.

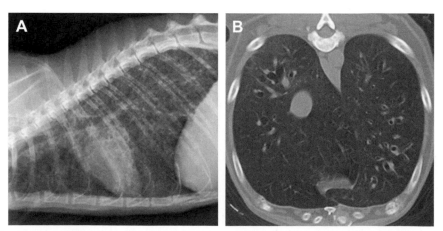

Fig. 12. Lateral thoracic radiographs of a 15-year-old, neutered, female, domestic shorthair cat (*A*) and thoracic CT scan of a 12-year-old, neutered female, Labrador retriever (*B*). In both cases, note the bronchocentric distribution of the increased opacity that forms an excessive number of enlarged lines and rings, especially near the periphery of the lungs.

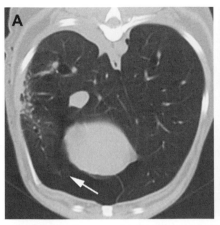
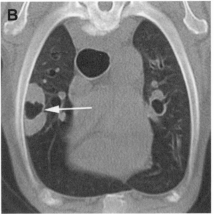

Fig. 13. Thoracic CT scans of a 7-year-old, neutered male poodle (*A*) with pneumothorax and a bleb (*arrow*) and of a 12-year-old, neutered female, Labrador retriever (*B*) with a cavity (*arrow*) in a soft-tissue mass (additional images of this dog are in **Fig. 11**).

CLINICAL INTEGRATION

The above Roentgen signs of altered opacity, degree of expansion, macroscopic distribution of the lesion, and appearance of the opacity may be combined to form radiographic patterns of lung disease. Some examples of radiographic patterns of lung disease are listed.

- Cranioventral air space pattern
- Consolidated lung lobe
- Caudodorsal-to-diffuse air space pattern
- Diffuse bronchocentric pattern
- Focal lung nodule (soft tissue)
- Multifocal lung nodules (soft tissue)

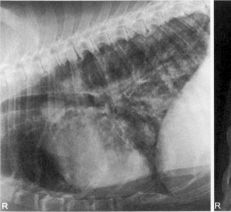
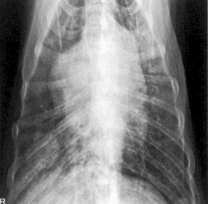

Fig. 14. Orthogonal thoracic radiographs of a 12-year-old, neutered, female German shepherd dog. Note the mixed-lung pattern, which is composed of an increased opacity that is diffuse bronchocentric and multifocal nodular (soft-tissue).

- Focal bleb or bulla
- Multifocal blebs or bullae
- Focal lung cavity
- Multifocal lung cavities
- Diffuse hyperlucent lung pattern
- Atelectasis (regional)
- Atelectasis (diffuse)
- Asymmetric air space pattern
- Mixed lung pattern

Suggested differential diagnoses for some of these patterns are available.[17,18] For example, the differential diagnosis for a cranioventral air space pattern includes aspiration or bronchopneumonia, hemorrhage, or cancer. The differential diagnosis for a caudodorsal-to-diffuse air space pattern includes such things as congestive left heart failure, toxin inhalation, some viral or parasitic infections, strangulation, near drowning, fibrosis, thermal injury, septicemia and endotoxemia, disseminated intravascular coagulation, and some cancers (eg, lymphoma). The differential diagnosis for a diffuse bronchocentric pattern includes all causes of bronchitis (eg, allergic, immune-mediated, infectious, viral, bacterial, parasitic), lymphatic spread of cancer, or early left-sided congestive heart failure. Differential diagnoses may be prioritized by incorporating other information such as signalment, history, and results of other tests.

Oftentimes, lung disease does not produce a radiographic pattern that can be neatly categorized, because there is a mixture of findings. Identifying a mixed pattern, however, is not helpful unless the different components are equally important. Most often, it is simply most efficacious to identify only the most important pattern, because that is what will help better define the cause of the problem. When multiple findings are equally important and it is appropriate to conclude a mixed pattern, then the disease may be due to one or multiple causes, and differential diagnoses for all patterns should be considered (**Fig. 14**).

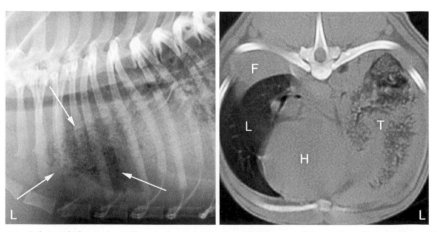

Fig. 15. A lateral thoracic radiograph and CT scan of a 3-year-old, neutered male Pug with a left-cranial-lung-lobe torsion. Note that the left-cranial lung lobe is fully expanded with locally extensive increased opacity that contains innumerable, small, gas bubbles (*arrows*, T). This combination of signs is consistent with lung-lobe torsion with lung necrosis. The heart (H), lung (L) and pleural fluid (F) also are indicated.

SUMMARY

It is important to acknowledge that the description in this article is incomplete. For example, the term *bronchiectasis*, which is irreversible, localized, or diffuse bronchial enlargement usually resulting from chronic infection, upstream airway obstruction, or congenital bronchial abnormality, was not mentioned.[20] Also, diseases that produce mineralization were not discussed. Therefore, the previous description should be considered as a starting point that may be useful for diagnosing commonly encountered pulmonary diseases. There are other signs (eg, bronchial foreign body) or patterns of lung disease that were not described and necessary to make other diagnoses. For example, a pattern of a fully expanded lung lobe with increased opacity that obscures pulmonary blood vessels and contains multiple gas bubbles may be observed in some dogs and cats with lung-lobe torsion; signs of pleural fluid may also be present **(Fig. 15)**.[18,26]

Pulmonary radiography is a complex process that is most effective when it combines clinical experience with scientific knowledge and is able to change with newly gathered information. Additionally, there is a need for radiologists to seek evidence that the proposed methods (whether traditional or non-traditional) actually improve patient care.

REFERENCES

1. Suter PF, Chan KF. Disseminated pulmonary diseases in small animals: a radiographic approach to diagnosis. Vet Radiol Ultrasound 1968;9:67–79.
2. Lord PF, Suter PF, Chan PF, et al. Pleural, extrapleural and pulmonary lesions in small animals: a radiographic approach to differential diagnosis. Vet Radiol Ultrasound 1972;13:4–17.
3. Myer W, Burt JK. Bronchiectasis in the dog: its radiographic appearance. Vet Radiol Ultrasound 1973;14:3–12.
4. Suter PF, Carrig CB, O'Brien TR, et al. Radiographic recognition of primary and metastatic pulmonary neoplasm of dogs and cats. Vet Radiol Ultrasound 1974; 15:3–24.
5. Myer W, Burt JK, Davis GW. A comparative study of propyliodone and barium bronchography in the dog. Vet Radiol Ultrasound 1974;15:44–55.
6. Silverman S, Poulos PW, Suter PF. Cavitary pulmonary lesions in animals. Vet Radiol Ultrasound 1976;17:134–46.
7. Myer W. Pneumothorax: a radiography review. Vet Radiol Ultrasound 1978;19: 12–5.
8. Myer W. Radiography review: pleural effusion. Vet Radiol Ultrasound 1978;19: 75–9.
9. Myer W. Radiography review: the extrapleural space. Vet Radiol Ultrasound 1978; 19:157–60.
10. Myer W. Radiography review: the mediastinum. Vet Radiol Ultrasound 1978;19: 197–202.
11. Myer W. Radiography review: the alveolar pattern of pulmonary disease. Vet Radiol Ultrasound 1979;20:10–4.
12. Myer W. Radiography review: the interstitial pattern of pulmonary disease. Vet Radiol Ultrasound 1980;21:18–23.
13. Myer CW. Radiography review: the vascular and bronchial patterns of pulmonary disease. Vet Radiol Ultrasound 1980;21:156–60.
14. Spencer CP, Ackerman N, Burt JK. The canine lateral thoracic radiograph. Vet Radiol Ultrasound 1981;22:262–6.

15. Suter PF. Thoracic radiography: a text atlas of thoracic diseases of the dog and cat. Wettswil: PF Suter; 1984. p. 517–682.
16. Lord PF, Gomez JA. Lung lobe collapse. Vet Radiol Ultrasound 1985;26:187–95.
17. Nykamp S, Scrivani PV, Dykes NL. Radiographic signs of pulmonary disease: an alternative approach. Compendium on Continuing Education for the Practicing Veterinarian 2002;24:25–36.
18. Maï W, O'Brien R, Scrivani P, et al. The lung parenchyma. In: Schwarz T, Johnson V, editors. BSAVA manual of canine and feline thoracic imaging. Gloucester: BSAVA; 2008. p. 258–60.
19. Winegardner KR, Scrivani PV, Gleed RD. Lung expansion in the diagnosis of lung disease. Compendium 2008;30:479–89.
20. Hansell DM, Bankier AA, MacMahon H, et al. Fleischner society: glossary of terms for thoracic imaging. Radiology 2008;246:697–721.
21. Wilcox JR. The written radiology report. Appl Radiol 2006;35:33–7.
22. Reed JC. Chest radiology: plain film patterns and differential diagnoses. 4th edition. St. Louis (MO): Mosby-Year Book; 1997. p. 185–432.
23. Lynch DA, Travis WD, Müller NL, et al. Idiopathic interstitial pneumonias: CT features. Radiology 2005;236:10–21.
24. Felson B. A new look at pattern recognition and diffuse pulmonary disease. Am J Roentgenol 1979;133:183–9.
25. McLoud TC, Carrington CB, Gaensler EA. Diffuse infiltrative lung disease: a new scheme for description. Radiology 1983;149:353–63.
26. D'Anjou MA, Tidwell AS, Hecht S. Radiographic diagnosis of lung lobe torsion. Vet Radiol Ultrasound 2005;46:478–84.

Ultrasound of the Thorax (Noncardiac)

Martha Moon Larson, DVM, MS

KEYWORDS

• Ultrasound • Thorax • Pleural effusion • Mediastinum • Lung

Ultrasound of the noncardiac thorax is an important supplemental imaging modality in the diagnosis of pulmonary, mediastinal, pleural, and chest wall disease. There are limitations, as there is near-total reflection of sound waves at gas interfaces, hiding pulmonary or mediastinal lesions located deep to the air-filled lung. However, if pulmonary lesions are peripheral, or pleural fluid is present to act as an acoustic window, ultrasound detection of disease is possible. The use of ultrasound to guide thoracocentesis, aspiration of masses, or lung consolidation increases efficiency and safety.

TECHNIQUE

Thoracic radiographs should always be taken before the ultrasound examination to assess disease and to determine the most appropriate scanning window. If pleural effusion is present, and the patient is stable, thoracocentesis should be delayed until after the ultrasound examination. Pleural fluid provides a valuable acoustic window to the lungs and mediastinum. Patients can be scanned in lateral or sternal recumbency, using an intercostal window. Dorsal recumbency may also be used if the patient is stable. Some patients may be more comfortable when scanned while standing. Both longitudinal (transducer perpendicular to ribs) and transverse (transducer parallel to ribs) imaging planes should be used. Lesions in the caudal thorax or mediastinum can be visualized using a transhepatic approach from a ventral or lateral abdominal location. A window through the thoracic inlet may allow enhanced visualization of the cranial mediastinum. A small footprint transducer (sector, curved microconvex, or curved linear array) fits best in restricted intercostal spaces. Transducer frequency should be based on the size of the patient and depth of the lesion.

NORMAL APPEARANCE

The chest wall is composed of skin, subcutaneous fat, and muscle. These tissues are represented by alternating layers of hyper- and hypoechogenicity in the near field, just

Department of Small Animal Clinical Sciences, Virginia-Maryland Regional College of Veterinary Medicine, Virginia Tech University, Duckpond Drive, Phase II, Blacksburg, VA 24061, USA
E-mail address: moonm@vt.edu

Vet Clin Small Anim 39 (2009) 733–745
doi:10.1016/j.cvsm.2009.04.006
0195-5616/09/$ – see front matter © 2009 Elsevier Inc. All rights reserved.

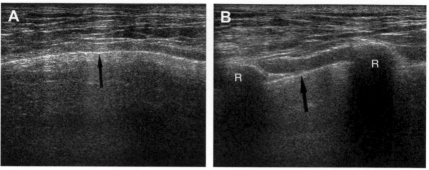

Fig. 1. (*A*) Transverse ultrasound scan of a normal thorax. The transducer is parallel to the ribs at the right seventh intercostal space. The chest wall is represented by alternating layers of hyper- and hypoechogenicity in the near field. The pleura-lung interface is represented by a smooth, linear echogenic line extending across the image (*arrow*). Dorsal is at the right side of the image. (*B*) Longitudinal ultrasound scan of a normal thorax. The transducer is aligned perpendicular to the ribs at the right seventh intercostal space. Ribs (R) are seen in cross section, creating a curvilinear echogenic interface with distal shadowing. The lung-pleura interface is represented by the smooth echogenic line between ribs (*arrow*). Cranial is to the left of the image.

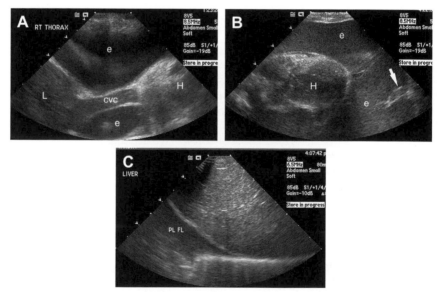

Fig. 2. (*A*) Longitudinal ultrasound scan of the caudal thorax in a dog with pleural effusion. The transducer is perpendicular to the ribs. Pleural effusion is present in both hemithoraces (e). The caudal vena cava (cvc) is seen extending from the liver (L) to the heart (H). Caudal is to the left of the image. (*B*) Longitudinal ultrasound scan of the caudal thorax of a cat with pleural effusion. The transducer is perpendicular to the ribs. Echogenic effusion (e) is seen in both hemithoraces. The heart (H) is seen cranially (to the left of the image). An echogenic fibrin strand is present caudally (*arrow*). Carcinomatosis was diagnosed on cytology of the pleural fluid. Note that this image is oriented the opposite of **Fig. 2***A*. (*C*) Longitudinal scan of the cranial abdomen of a dog with pleural effusion. Pleural fluid (PL FL) is seen cranial to the diaphragm, with the liver located caudally. A transhepatic window is used to detect the pleural fluid. Cranial is to the left of the image.

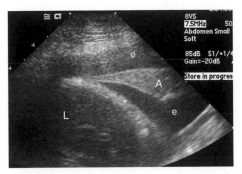

Fig. 3. Longitudinal ultrasound scan of a dog with pleural effusion. Pleural fluid (e) surrounds a small, triangular hypoechoic collapsed lung lobe (A). The liver (L) is seen caudally (to the left of the image).

beneath the transducer (**Fig. 1**).[1–5] The parietal pleura lining the thoracic wall may not be seen distinctly, and in the normal dog and cat, the visceral pleura and lung surface form a continuous echogenic line. However, the two pleural interfaces may be differentiated by the "gliding sign," with the hyperechoic pleuropulmonary interface moving smoothly during respiration against the parietal pleura lining the chest wall.[1,2,5,6] Normal lung tissue deep to the visceral pleural interface is obscured by shadowing and reverberation artifact. Ribs are represented by smooth curvilinear echogenic interfaces with acoustic shadowing and are seen in regular intervals as the chest wall is scanned.

PLEURAL DISEASE

Thoracic ultrasound provides reliable determination of the presence, volume, and characteristics of pleural fluid.[1–5] Pleural fluid creates an excellent acoustic window, allowing ultrasound visualization of intrathoracic anatomy, including pulmonary, chest wall, and mediastinal disease not visible radiographically (**Fig. 2**). The fluid will appear anechoic if it is a transudate, modified transudate, or chylous effusion. The fluid will appear echogenic if there are cells, fibrin, and/or protein (exudates, hemorrhage, or neoplastic effusions) within the fluid. Pleural fluid accumulates between the thoracic wall and diaphragm, surrounding and extending between lung lobes. Small or localized fluid pockets may be more difficult to see, and accompanying thoracic radiographs should always be taken to help pinpoint the location of smaller quantities of

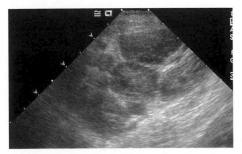

Fig. 4. Longitudinal ultrasound scan of the cranial mediastinum in a dog. A cranial mediastinal mass is seen, appearing as a coalescing mass of hypoechoic nodules. Lymphosarcoma was diagnosed on cytology from a fine-needle aspirate of the mass. Cranial is to the left of the image.

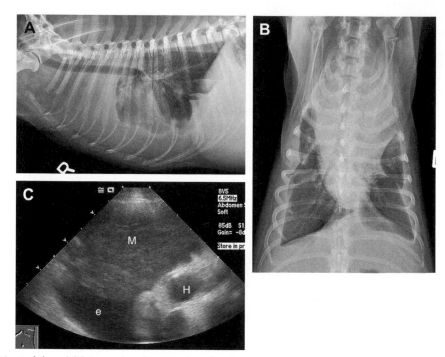

Fig. 5. (*A*) and (*B*) Lateral and ventrodorsal radiographs of a dog presented for respiratory distress. Pleural effusion is present, along with a widened cranial mediastinum seen best on the ventrodorsal view. (*C*) Transverse ultrasound image of the right thoracic wall of the dog in **Figs. 5** *A* and *B*. A large, homogeneous, hypoechoic mass (M) is seen adjacent to the heart (H). Pleural effusion (e) is seen ventral to the mass. A thymoma was diagnosed on cytology of the mass obtained on fine-needle aspiration Dorsal is at the right side of the image.

pleural fluid. In these cases, scanning the dependent thoracic region aids in fluid visualization. Pleural thickening, represented by a roughened, irregular surface lining the thoracic wall, may indicate pleuritis, neoplastic pleural disease, or chronic effusions. Echogenic linear fibrin strands are frequently seen with chronic effusion. Masses involving the pleura can be differentiated from pulmonary masses by the more peripheral location and lack of movement. Pulmonary masses will move with the lungs during respiration. As pleural fluid accumulates, lung lobes will collapse, forming small, wedge-shaped, or triangular structures (**Fig. 3**). With complete collapse, the shrunken lobes will be completely hypoechoic and appear to float within the surrounding pleural fluid. Although the cause of the pleural effusion may not always be apparent, a complete search of the thoracic wall, heart, lungs, and diaphragm should always be performed. Thoracic ultrasound can also be used in the diagnosis of pneumothorax and may be helpful as a quick initial screening tool in severely dyspneic or stressed patients.[6] Pneumothorax is diagnosed when the normal gliding sign between pleural margins cannot be seen. The glide sign indicates normal apposition of lung against the thoracic wall and is not present with pneumothorax.[1,2,5,6]

CRANIAL MEDIASTINUM

A parasternal or thoracic inlet approach is best for evaluating the cranial mediastinal area. Although normal mediastinal tissues can be seen in some patients, pleural effusion creates a more effective ultrasound window to see mediastinal anatomy (**Fig. 2A**).[1–4] Large anechoic vessels extend cranially toward the thoracic inlet and may be surrounded by varying amounts of echogenic and irregular mediastinal fat. This normal fat should not be confused with a true mass, which is typically better marginated and may cause displacement of adjacent structures. Ultrasound is very helpful in differentiating a true mediastinal mass from normal fat in patients with a widened mediastinum on thoracic radiographs. The thymus may be visualized as a granular, coarse echogenic structure ventral to the mediastinal vessels in young dogs and cats.[1] Normal mediastinal and sternal lymph nodes are not typically seen. Detection of mediastinal masses depends on the size and location.[1–7] Large masses that extend to the thoracic wall are easily seen. Smaller masses require the presence of pleural effusion to act as an acoustic window for detection. Mediastinal masses are found most commonly in the cranioventral mediastinum and are located primarily on the midline. Frequently these masses are diffusely hypoechoic and lobular (lymph node origin) or may have more complex heterogeneous or cystic structures (**Figs. 4 and 5**). Mediastinal masses are often accompanied by pleural effusion. Neoplastic lesions of the mediastinum, including lymphosarcoma, thymoma, neuroendocrine tumors, lymphomatoid granulomatosis, mast cell tumor, melanoma, and thyroid carcinoma, should all be considered, and the ultrasound appearance alone is insufficient for complete diagnosis (**Fig. 6**).[1–7] Mediastinal granulomas, hematomas, and abscesses occur less commonly but can appear identical to neoplastic masses.

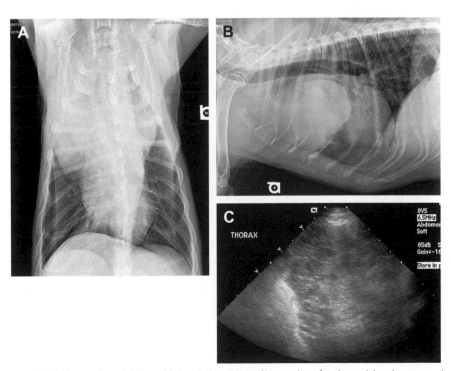

Fig. 6. (*A, B*) Ventrodorsal (*A*) and lateral thoracic radiographs of a dog with a large cranial mediastinal mass. (*C*) Transverse ultrasound image of the cranial mediastinal area of the dog in **Figs. 6** *A* and *B*. A large, heterogeneous mass is seen. The mass is hyperechoic, with multiple hypoechoic nodules distributed throughout. Dorsal is at the right side of the image.

Idiopathic mediastinal cysts have been reported in geriatric cats.[8] These cysts are typically ovoid to bi-lobed in shape, with a well-marginated echogenic wall surrounding anechoic fluid (**Fig. 7**). Clear fluid with a low cell count is noted on cyst aspiration. Thymomas may also have a cystic appearance but should be thicker and more irregular. Heart base tumors, although more centrally located, can be visualized using the heart as an acoustic window. Caudal esophageal masses may be seen from a transhepatic approach. Ultrasound-guided aspiration or biopsy of mediastinal mass is essential in establishing a more definitive diagnosis and is critical when lesions are small or surrounded by adjacent vessels.

PULMONARY DISEASE

The lung parenchyma can be evaluated with ultrasound if air has been removed (atelectasis) or replaced by fluid or cells (the same process that results in increased radiographic opacity of lungs). However, the diseased lung must either extend to the lung periphery or be surrounded by fluid. Any aerated lung between the transducer and lesion is sufficient to mask the lung abnormality.

LUNG CONSOLIDATION

Infiltrative disease of the lung will cause an interruption in the echogenic linear lung interface, with hypoechoic tissue replacing air-filled lung.[1–5] With early or mild disease,

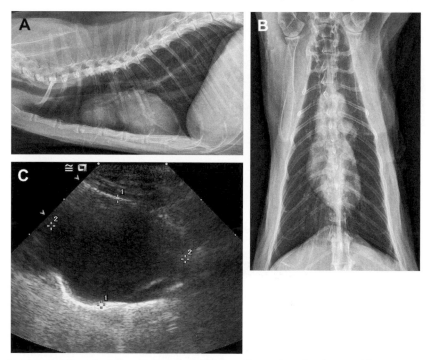

Fig. 7. Lateral (A) and ventrodorsal (B) thoracic radiographs of a 9-year-old cat. A cranial mediastinal mass is noted just cranial to the heart on the lateral view. This mass causes widening of the cranial mediastinum on the ventrodorsal view. (C) Longitudinal ultrasound image of the right cranial thoracic wall of the cat in **Figs. 7** A and B. An anechoic, well-defined cystic structure is seen (between calipers). A clear transudate was removed on aspiration, and a benign mediastinal cyst was diagnosed. Cranial is to the left of the image.

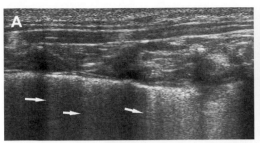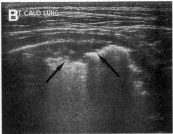

Fig. 8. (A) Longitudinal ultrasound image of the right thoracic wall in a dog presented for coughing. The normal linear echogenic lung/pleura interface is interrupted by numerous echogenic foci with hyperechoic shadows (*arrows*). These are termed comet tails and can indicate early pulmonary infiltrative disease. Cranial is to the left of the image. (B) Longitudinal ultrasound image of the right thoracic wall in a dog with pneumonia. A focal peripheral section of lung is hypoechoic due to fluid replacing normal aerated tissue (*arrows*). Normal air-filled lung is displaced deeper into the image. Cranial is to the left.

this interruption of the lung interface is seen as small hyperechoic foci with distal shadowing, termed comet tails (or perhaps, more correctly, ring-down artifact).[9,10] These artifacts are nonspecific and can be seen with pulmonary edema, pleuritis, pulmonary fibrosis, interstitial pneumonia, and pulmonary contusion, diseases characterized by a thickening of either the pleura or the interlobular septa (**Fig. 8**).[9,10] As the disease process becomes more extensive, aerated lung is displaced further and further from the chest wall. Although relatively homogeneous and hypoechoic, the diseased lung will also contain hyperechoic, shadowing linear structures resulting from residual air in the bronchi (air bronchograms), as well as more punctate echogenic foci from remaining air-filled alveoli (**Fig. 9**).[1–5] Fluid-filled bronchi may also be seen and can be differentiated from pulmonary vessels only by Doppler interrogation. When severe lung consolidation is present, the echogenicity and texture are similar to that of the liver, and this condition is termed hepatization (**Fig. 10**).[1–5] Lung consolidation can occur with pneumonia, edema, lung lobe torsion, contusions, and some lobar neoplasias.[1] With consolidation, the lung retains its normal volume, unlike atelectasis, which appears similar in echogenicity and texture but is decreased in volume. Lung lobe torsions will appear as a consolidated lobe on thoracic ultrasound, usually surrounded by pleural effusion (**Fig. 11**). The affected lung lobe can appear hypoechoic at the

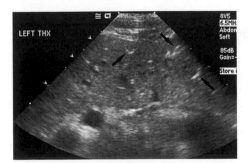

Fig. 9. Transverse ultrasound image of the left thoracic wall in a dog with severe pneumonia. A large segment of lung is consolidated and hypoechoic. Multiple air bronchograms are seen as hyperechoic linear structures (*arrows*). Dorsal is at the top of the image.

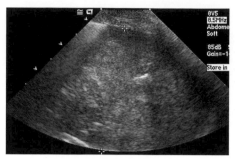

Fig. 10. Longitudinal ultrasound image of the right thoracic wall in a dog with severe pneumonia. The lung lobe (between calipers) has an echogenicity and texture similar to the liver, termed "hepatization." Cranial is to the left of the image.

periphery but centrally may contain multiple echogenic foci representing gas **(Fig. 12)**.[11] This gas is consistent with the vesicular gas patterns often seen on radiographs. The torsed lobe will be normal to increased in volume, may have rounded margins, and extend in an abnormal position. Typically, there is no venous signal when lobar vessels are examined with Doppler. In some cases, a faint arterial signal may still be present.

PULMONARY MASSES

Neoplastic pulmonary disease results in homogeneous or heterogeneous lung masses that may have a smoother deep margin compared with the more irregular lung margin often seen with non-neoplastic consolidations **(Figs. 13 and 14)**.[1–5] There may be

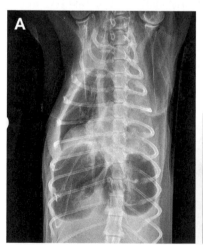

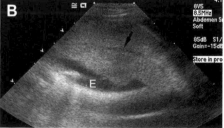

Fig. 11. (A) Ventrodorsal thoracic radiograph of an 8-year-old cat presented for respiratory distress. Pleural effusion, along with increased opacity of the right middle lung lobe is noted. (B) Longitudinal ultrasound image of the right thoracic wall of the cat in **Fig. 11**A. The right middle lung lobe is surrounded by pleural effusion (E) and is completely hypoechoic. The volume does not appear reduced, and the lobe maintains a normal shape. A fluid bronchogram runs down the middle of the lobe (*arrow*). Right middle lobe lung torsion was diagnosed at necropsy. Cranial is to the left of the image.

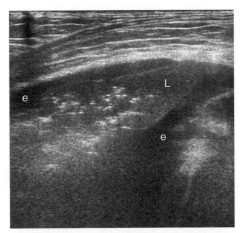

Fig. 12. Longitudinal ultrasound image of the right thoracic wall of a dog with lung lobe torsion. The torsed lobe (L) is surrounded by pleural effusion (e). The periphery of the lobe is hypoechoic, whereas the more central portion contains multiple echogenic foci representing gas. Cranial is to the left of the image.

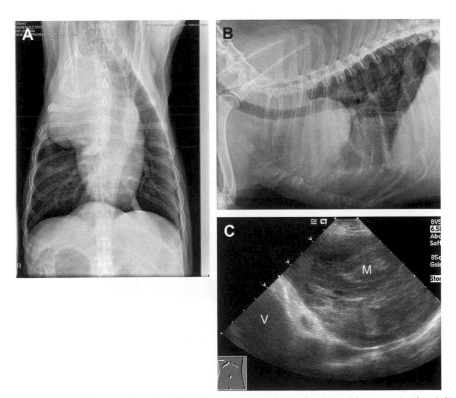

Fig. 13. (A) and (B) Ventrodorsal and left lateral radiograph of a dog with a mass in the right cranial lung lobe. (C) Longitudinal ultrasound image of the right thoracic wall of the dog in **Fig. 13**. A large heterogeneous mass (M) with some anechoic areas is present between the right thoracic wall and the right side of the heart (V). Pulmonary adenocarcinoma was diagnosed on cytology from a fine-needle aspirate. Cranial is to the left of the image.

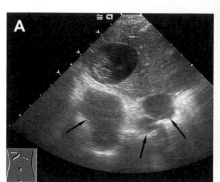
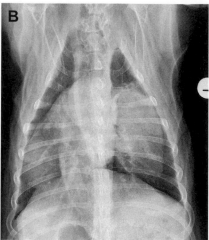

Fig. 14. (*A*) Transverse ultrasound image of the liver in an 11-year-old dog. This image was made from the ventral abdomen, just caudal to the xiphoid. Multiple hypoechoic nodules are visible cranial to the diaphragm (*arrows*). Ventral is at the top of the image, with right side at the left of the image. (*B*) Ventrodorsal radiograph of the dog in **Fig. 14***A*. Large soft tissue masses are noted in the right middle, accessory, and left cranial (caudal segment) lung lobes. This dog did not present for respiratory signs, and thoracic radiographs were taken only after pulmonary masses were seen on abdominal ultrasound. Pulmonary carcinoma was diagnosed on cytology from fine-needle aspiration.

a distinct delineation between normal aerated lung and pulmonary mass. If pleural effusion surrounds the affected lung, the mass can be seen to bulge from or deform the lobe (**Fig. 15**). A uniform hypoechogenicity identical to lung consolidation (eg, pneumonia) may be present, and biopsy or fine-needle aspiration is necessary for a definitive diagnosis. Small pulmonary nodules such as fungal granulomas or metastatic disease, if peripheral, create well-demarcated, spherical mass lesions (**Fig. 16**). Like all pulmonary origin masses, they move with respiration.

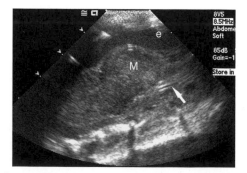

Fig. 15. Longitudinal ultrasound image of the right thoracic wall of a cat presented for respiratory distress. Pleural effusion (*e*) surrounds a collapsed right cranial lung lobe. A fluid bronchogram extends through the lobe (*arrow*). A mass (*M*) bulges from the lung margin. Pulmonary carcinoma was diagnosed on cytology from fine-needle aspiration. Cranial is to the left of the image.

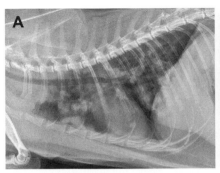 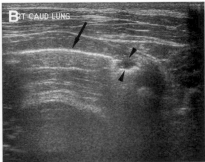

Fig. 16. (A) Lateral thoracic radiograph of a cat presented for mild respiratory distress. Multiple soft tissue nodules are present. (B) Longitudinal ultrasound image of the right thoracic wall of the cat in Fig. 16A. A normal lung/pleura interface is seen cranially (*arrow*) but is interrupted caudally by a small spherical hypoechoic nodule (*arrowheads*). Blastomycosis was diagnosed on cytology from fine-needle aspiration. Cranial is to the left of the image.

ATELECTASIS

Atelectasis secondary to pleural effusion is seen readily on ultrasound examination. The lung lobes decrease in volume, forming small triangular structures surrounded by fluid (see Fig. 3).[1–5] Residual alveolar and bronchial air will form multifocal echogenic linear structures (air bronchograms) and foci. With complete collapse, the lobe will be uniformly hypoechoic. Atelectasis secondary to pneumothorax cannot be visualized with ultrasound due to surrounding air interfaces.

DIAPHRAGMATIC HERNIA

Radiographic diagnosis of diaphragmatic hernias can be challenging. Pleural effusion can obscure visualization of herniated abdominal viscera, or these displaced organs could mimic a pulmonary mass. Ultrasound examination, using left and right intercostal (5th–13th intercostal spaces) and transhepatic windows, can be a valuable adjunct imaging modality.[1–5,12] The normal diaphragm (actually the diaphragm/lung interface) is visualized as a curvilinear echogenic band surrounding the cranial margin

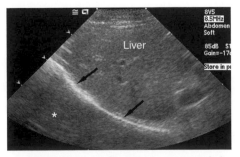

Fig. 17. Longitudinal ultrasound image of the liver in a normal dog. The diaphragm/lung interface is represented by a curvilinear echogenic line along the cranial margin of the liver (*arrows*). A mirror image artifact (*) creates the appearance of the liver cranial to the diaphragm. Cranial is to the left of the image, with ventral at the top.

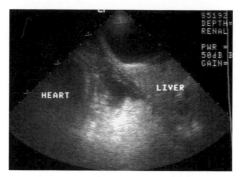

Fig. 18. Longitudinal ultrasound image of the cranial abdomen in a dog with a diaphragmatic hernia. The normal echogenic linear diaphragm/lung interface is no longer present along the cranial margin of the liver. Anechoic pleural effusion separates the cranially displaced liver from the heart. On abdominal exploration, the liver was found to be herniated above the diaphragm.

of the liver (**Fig. 17**). The true diaphragm is seen as a separate echogenic line if pleural and peritoneal effusion are present. Frequently, a mirror image artifact is present in normal dogs, giving the impression of liver on both sides of the diaphragm. The diaphragm must be intact for this artifact to occur, so recognition of this phenomenon should help to rule out a true diaphragmatic hernia in that area. Discontinuity of the diaphragm or an irregular or asymmetric cranial hepatic margin is a common finding with a diaphragmatic hernia. Cranial displacement of abdominal viscera confirms the diagnosis (**Fig. 18**). Displaced abdominal organs are usually seen lateral to the heart. It is important to differentiate consolidated lung tissue (hepatization) from the true liver. Multiple windows, both intercostal and transhepatic, are necessary for evaluation of the entire diaphragm.

Pericardial-peritoneal diaphragmatic hernias (PPDH) are congenital defects that result in varying amounts of abdominal viscera or omentum cranially displaced into the pericardial sac. Generalized cardiomegaly is typically present on thoracic radiographs. Thoracic ultrasound, using either an intercostal or cardiac window, can be used to differentiate PPDH from acquired and congenital primary heart disease. Abdominal viscera, such as liver, will surround the heart and be contained within the pericardial sac. If only a small amount of falciform fat is herniated, diagnosis becomes much more difficult. Again, a careful search for discontinuity of the diaphragm is necessary.

SUMMARY

Thoracic ultrasound is an extremely valuable imaging modality for diseases of the pleura, mediastinum, lungs, and chest wall. Pleural effusion, often a detriment for radiographic evaluation of thoracic structures, provides an excellent window for ultrasound visualization of thoracic anatomy. Ultrasound-guided aspirate/biopsy allows minimally invasive collection of cytology or histopathology for diagnosis of thoracic pathology.

REFERENCES

1. Mattoon JS, Nyland TG. Thorax. In: Nyland TG, Mattoon J, editors. Small animal diagnostic ultrasound. 2nd edition. Philadelphia: WB Saunders; 2002. p. 325–53.

2. Hecht S. Thorax. In: Penninck D, D'Anjoy MA, editors. Atlas of small animal ultrasonography. Ames (IA): Blackwell Publishing; 2008. p. 119–50.
3. Reichle JK, Wisner ER. Non-cardiac thoracic ultrasound in 75 feline and canine patients. Vet Radiol Ultrasound 2000;41:154–62.
4. Stowater JL, Lamb CR. Ultrasonography of noncardiac thoracic diseases in small animals. J Am Vet Med Assoc 1989;195:514–20.
5. Saunders HM, Keith D. Thoracic imaging. In: King LG, editor. Textbook of respiratory diseases in dogs and cats. Philadelphia: WB Saunders; 2004. p. 72–93.
6. Lisciandro GR, Lagutchik MS, Mann KA, et al. Evaluation of a thoracic focused assessment with sonography for trauma (TFAST) protocol to detect pneumothorax and concurrent thoracic injury in 145 traumatized dogs. J Vet Emerg Crit Care 2008;18:258–69.
7. Konde LJ, Spaulding K. Sonographic evaluation of the cranial mediastinum in small animals. Vet Radiol 1991;32:178–84.
8. Zekas LJ, Adams WM. Cranial mediastinal cysts in nine cats. Vet Radiol Ultrasound 2002;43:413–8.
9. ReiBig A, Kroegel C. Transthoracic sonography of diffuse parenchymal lung disease. J Ultrasound Med 2003;22:173–80.
10. Louvet A, Bourgeois JM. Lung ring-down artifact as a sign of pulmonary alveolar-interstitial disease. Vet Radiol Ultrasound 2008;49:374–7.
11. D'Anjou MA, Tidwell AS, Hecht S. Radiographic diagnosis of lung lobe torsion. Vet Radiol Ultrasound 2005;46:478–84.
12. Spattini G, Rossi F, Vignoli M, et al. Use of ultrasound to diagnose diaphragmatic rupture in dogs and cats. Vet Radiol Ultrasound 2003;44:226–30.

Ultrasound of the Gastrointestinal Tract

Martha Moon Larson, DVM, MS[a],*, David S. Biller, DVM[b]

KEYWORDS

- Ultrasound • Gastrointestinal tract • Enteritis
- Neoplasia • Obstruction

Familiarity with the normal and abnormal ultrasound appearance of the canine and feline gastrointestinal (GI) tract provides a marked advantage in the diagnosis of GI disease. Although gas may inhibit complete visualization, in many cases, ultrasound is able to confirm or rule out suspected disease. It should be noted that ultrasound of the GI tract does not preclude the need for abdominal radiographs. The two imaging modalities are complementary, and each adds individual information. Ultrasound evaluation of the GI tract provides information about bowel wall thickness and layers, assessment of motility, and visualization of important adjacent structures such as lymph nodes and peritoneum. In the hands of experienced sonographers, abdominal ultrasound has replaced the need for GI contrast studies in many cases, saving time, money, radiation exposure, and stress to the patient.

Techniques and approaches vary somewhat on patient conformation and position. Scanning the patient in dorsal recumbency allows relatively complete evaluation of the GI tract, although right and left lateral recumbency may be necessary to redistribute gas and fluid within individual portions of the stomach and bowel. Right lateral intercostal windows are often helpful in visualizing the pylorus and proximal duodenum in deep-chested dogs. Scanning the ventral abdomen of the standing dog or cat may allow improved visualization of the dependent pylorus and gastric body. In most patients, a high-frequency transducer (7.5 MHz or higher) is used for better visualization of stomach, small intestines, and colonic wall thickness and layers. A sector or curvilinear transducer is best for intercostal windows due to the smaller contact area of these probes.

The canine stomach can be accessed immediately caudal to the liver, at the level of the xiphoid. The feline gastric fundus and body are left-sided structures, with the pylorus located in a more midline location. In both species, the left-sided dorsal fundus should be followed ventrally and to the right, toward the pylorus, using both

[a] Department of Small Animal Clinical Sciences, Virginia-Maryland Regional College of Veterinary Medicine, Virginia Tech University, Duckpond Drive, Phase II, Blacksburg, VA 24061, USA
[b] Department of Clinical Sciences, Kansas State University, College of Veterinary Medicine, Veterinary Medical Teaching Hospital, 1800 Denison Avenue, Manhattan, KS 66506, USA
* Corresponding author.
E-mail address: moonm@vt.edu (M.M. Larson).

Vet Clin Small Anim 39 (2009) 747–759
doi:10.1016/j.cvsm.2009.04.010
0195-5616/09/$ – see front matter © 2009 Elsevier Inc. All rights reserved.

vetsmall.theclinics.com

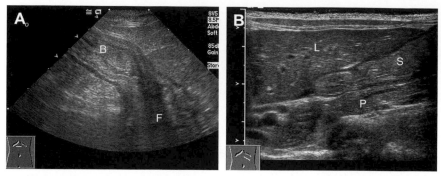

Fig.1. (A) Ultrasound image of the long axis view of the normal canine stomach. The fundus (F) is located dorsally and to the left, with the body (B) located more ventrally and to the right. Normal gastric wall layers are noted. Some echogenic fluid is within the gastric lumen. The body image in the lower left corner of the image demonstrates transducer position. Ventral is at the top of the image, with right side of the body at the left side of the image. (B) Ultrasound image of the long axis view of the normal feline stomach (S). The liver (L) is located immediately cranial to the stomach, with the left limb and body of the pancreas (P) located just caudal to the stomach. The body image in the lower left corner of the image demonstrates transducer position. Ventral is at the top of the image, with the right side of the body at the left side of the image.

longitudinal and transverse imaging planes (**Fig. 1**). In many patients, intraluminal gas allows visualization of only the near wall. Reverberation artifact and shadowing lie deep to the echogenic gas interface, masking the lumen and far walls. In non–deep-chested dogs, or dogs with hepatomegaly, the pylorus can often be followed into the proximal duodenum from the ventral abdominal window. In cats, all parts of the stomach, including the pyloric-duodenal junction, are commonly seen. The canine descending duodenum is consistently located along the right lateral abdominal wall, just ventral and either medial or lateral to the right kidney (**Fig. 2**). In the dog, the descending duodenum is larger in diameter and follows a more linear cranial to caudal path than the adjacent jejunal segments. The feline duodenum is located closer to the midline and is the same diameter as the jejunum. It may appear segmented, representing the "string of pearls" sign often noted on barium contrast studies. In both species,

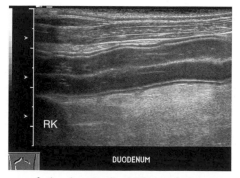

Fig. 2. Ultrasound image of the longitudinal view of the normal canine descending duodenum. The duodenum is located immediately ventral to the right kidney (RK) as it extends from cranial to caudal along the right lateral abdomen. Ventral is at the top of the image, with cranial on the left side of the image.

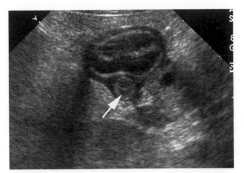

Fig. 3. Transverse image of the proximal duodenum at the level of the duodenal papilla. The bile duct (*arrow*) is visible entering the papilla. Ventral is at the top of the image, with the right on the left side of the image.

the duodenal papilla is visualized as a small focal nodule entering the proximal duodenum (**Fig. 3**).

Jejunal bowel loops are found throughout the abdomen. Although much of the jejunum can be seen while evaluating the major abdominal organs during the complete examination, a careful systematic scan over the mid-abdomen should be done for a more complete bowel examination.

In cats, the ileo-ceco-colic junction is consistently seen, just medial to the right kidney and adjacent to the colic lymph nodes. A smaller cecum, with less intraluminal gas, allows more consistent evaluation than in the dog, where cecal and colonic gas usually masks this area (**Fig. 4**).

The colon is usually the most difficult portion of the GI tract to evaluate due to intraluminal gas and fecal material. The transverse colon lies immediately caudal to the stomach. The descending colon can be followed caudally, where it lies just dorsal to the bladder (**Fig. 5**).

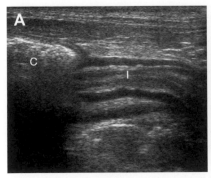
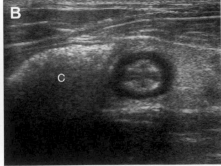

Fig. 4. (*A*) Longitudinal image of the normal feline ileo-colic junction. The terminal ileum (I) is seen entering the gas-filled colon (C). Ventral is at the top of the image, and cranial is to the left. (*B*) Transverse image of the normal feline terminal ileum just before it enters the gas-filled colon (C). Note the "wagon-wheel" appearance of the layers in the ileum. Ventral is at the top of the image, with the right on the left of the image.

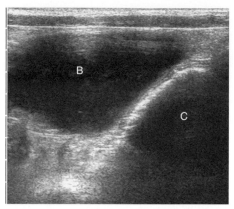

Fig. 5. Longitudinal image of the bladder (B) and descending colon (C). The gas-filled colon is normally seen just dorsal to the bladder in the caudal abdomen. Ventral is at the top of the image, with the cranial at the left.

NORMAL APPEARANCE

Five distinct layers are visible in the wall of the stomach and intestine (**Fig. 6**).[1–6] A bright hyperechoic mucosal-luminal interface is seen centrally. Peripheral to this interface is the hypoechoic mucosal layer, followed by a thin hyperechoic submucosa. Continuing peripherally is a thin hypoechoic muscularis layer, followed by the outermost hyperechoic serosa. The mucosal layer is normally thicker than the other layers in the small bowel. In the stomach, however, the muscularis layer is equal in thickness to the mucosal layer. Wall layers are best examined with a high-frequency transducer. Normal wall thicknesses for the intestines and stomach have been published (see **Table 1**).[1–6] In the dog, duodenal and jejunal thickness is dependent on body weight. All wall thickness measurements are taken from the inner mucosal interface to the outer aspect of the serosa (see **Fig. 6**). Wall thickness can be difficult to evaluate in the collapsed stomach, where the lumen is sometimes difficult to separate from the

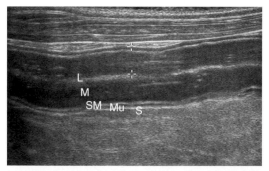

Fig. 6. Longitudinal image of the descending duodenum illustrating the individual wall layers. The hyperechoic mucosal-luminal interface (L) is centrally located and is followed by the prominent hypoechoic mucosal layer (M). The submucosa (SM) is a thin hyperechoic layer adjacent to the mucosa and is followed peripherally by the thin hypoechoic muscularis layer (Mu). Most peripheral is the thin hyperechoic serosal layer (S). Note the relative thickness of the layers; the mucosal layer is normally the thickest.

Table 1
Range of normal gastric and intestinal segment wall thicknesses

GI Segment	Canine (mm)	Feline (mm)
Stomach	3–5	1.1–3.6
Duodenum	2–6	1.3–3.8
Jejunum	2–4.7	1.5–3.6
Ileum		2.5–3.2
Colon		1.1–2.5

Data from Refs.[1–6]

wall. When gastric wall measurements are taken, it is important to measure between rugal folds to avoid artifactual increase in thickness. The normal but contracted stomach can also appear artifactually thickened.[7]

The stomach is occasionally empty but usually contains gas, fluid, or ingesta. Food aggregates appear as hypoechoic structures that move with peristalsis. Unlike true mass lesions, food does not persist when serial examinations are performed over time. When the stomach is empty, prominent rugal folds are visible. These are especially prominent in the cat, where they resemble spokes on a wheel (**Fig. 7**). The small intestines, usually empty, may also contain fluid or gas and, occasionally, ingesta. Fecal material and gas typically fill the colon, making wall measurements difficult. The terminal ileum in the cat is usually visible entering into the colon. The ileum has a more prominent muscularis and submucosa layer than other parts of the feline intestine and resembles a "wagon wheel" when seen in cross section (see **Fig. 4**).[6]

GI motility can be assessed by counting peristaltic waves. Typically, the stomach and small intestines undergo about three to five contractions per minute.[1]

ABNORMAL APPEARANCE

The stomach and bowel should be evaluated for wall thickness, appearance of wall layers, peristaltic activity, and luminal contents and diameter. Adjacent lymph nodes should be evaluated for enlargement, and the presence of free gas or fluid should be noted.

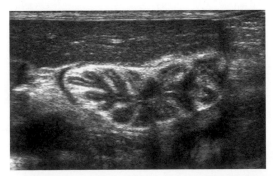

Fig. 7. Transverse image of the normal feline fundus. Note the prominent rugal folds resembling "spokes on a wheel." Ventral is at the top of the image, with the right side on the left of the image.

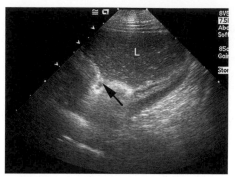

Fig. 8. Longitudinal image of the pyloric outflow area of a dog presenting with chronic vomiting. The pyloric outflow is markedly narrowed (*arrow*) by thickened pyloric walls. The lumen (L) caudal to the pylorus is distended with fluid. Lymphosarcoma was diagnosed with endoscopic biopsies.

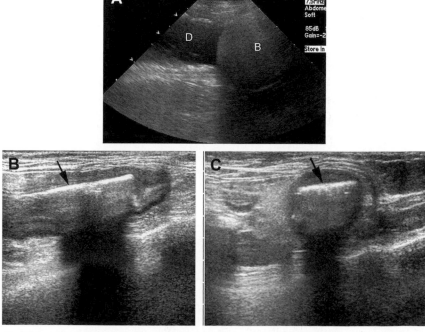

Fig. 9. (*A*) Longitudinal image of the descending duodenum. The duodenal lumen (D) is distended with fluid. An echogenic structure with round, well-defined margins (B) is obstructing the duodenum. A ball foreign body was removed surgically. Ventral is at the top of the image, with the cranial to the left. (*B*) Longitudinal and (*C*) cross-sectional images of the jejunum of a cat presented for vomiting. A well-defined linear echogenic structure (*arrows*) with acoustic shadowing is present within the jejunal lumen. This structure did not change in appearance or move with peristaltic activity. Plastic foreign material was removed surgically.

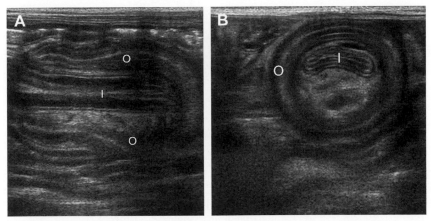

Fig. 10. Longitudinal (*A*) and cross-sectional (*B*) images of a jejunal intussusception in a puppy presented for vomiting. The intussusceptiens (O) are located outside the inner intussusceptum (I). Hyperechoic mesenteric fat is present adjacent to the intussusceptum.

OBSTRUCTION

Ultrasound examination is very helpful in determining if a pyloric or intestinal obstruction is present, and, when performed by an experienced sonographer, may replace a contrast GI series for confirmation of obstruction.[3,4,8,9] The actual cause of the obstruction may be better visualized on ultrasound examination than abdominal radiographs. Pyloric outflow obstruction, especially if chronic, usually results in fluid distension of the gastric lumen. The fluid enhances visualization of the pylorus and any potential foreign bodies or wall thickening (**Fig. 8**). The same is true of the small intestine, and any luminal distension should be followed to determine if an obstructive lesion is present. The appearance of a foreign body varies depending on the composition.[3,4,8–10] Some foreign objects, such as some types of balls, have through transmission, permitting visualization of the actual shape and size. However, many foreign bodies result only in a bright echogenic interface with acoustic shadowing. Only the near surface is visible and may have an irregular or more linear or curvilinear shape

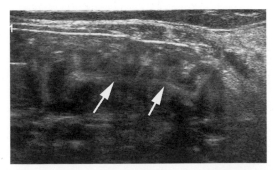

Fig. 11. Longitudinal image of a segment of jejunum in a cat presented for vomiting. The bowel segment is severely plicated, with a persistent linear echogenic structure extending through the lumen (*arrows*). A linear foreign body was removed surgically.

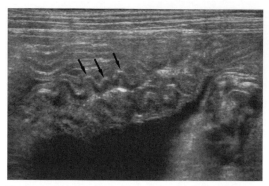

Fig. 12. Longitudinal image of a segment of jejunum in a dog with uroabdomen. Anechoic free fluid surrounds a segment of corrugated jejunum. Note the "rippled" appearance of the bowel, most apparent in the hyperechoic submucosal layer (*arrows*).

that usually takes the shape of the foreign material (**Fig. 9**). The bowel proximal (orad) to the obstruction is usually dilated with either gas or fluid.

INTUSSUSCEPTIONS

Ultrasound is an excellent imaging modality for the diagnosis of intussusceptions, as they are easily visualized and characteristic in appearance. When seen in cross section, the multiple bowel wall layers involved result in a bull's-eye or target-like appearance (repeated concentric rings).[3,4,9–13] These same multiple layers aligned in a parallel fashion are seen in longitudinal image planes (**Fig. 10**). Mesenteric fat is often carried in along with the intussusceptum (inner bowel loop), creating a bright, hyperechoic signal around the intussuscepted bowel segment. There is usually dilation of the section of the bowel orad to the intussusception.

LINEAR FOREIGN BODIES

Linear foreign bodies may also be identified on ultrasound examination.[3,4,9] The affected segment of bowel appears plicated or bunched, just as it does on abdominal radiographs. A persistent echogenic linear structure is often seen extending through the plicated bowel, representing the linear foreign material (**Fig. 11**). This linear

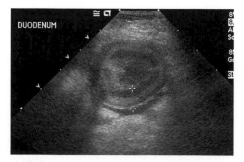

Fig. 13. Transverse image of the proximal duodenum in a dog with severe pancreatitis. The duodenal layers are maintained but have lost some of their definition secondary to inflammation. Compare this image of the duodenum to the normal transverse image in **Fig. 3**.

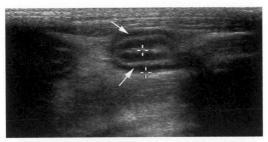

Fig. 14. Transverse image of a segment of jejunum in a cat with inflammatory bowel disease. The muscularis layer (*arrows*) is prominent and equal in thickness to the mucosal layer. The overall bowel wall thickness (*between calipers*) was increased at 3.5 mm.

echogenic structure does not change appearance or move with peristalsis. The stomach should always be checked for an anchoring portion of the linear foreign body, if not found under the tongue. Intussusceptions may occur secondary to linear foreign bodies and may be found in addition to plicated bowel. Corrugation of bowel, with a characteristic "rippling" of the submucosal layer, is seen with inflammation and should not be confused with intestinal plication (**Fig. 12**).

INFILTRATIVE DISEASE

The ultrasound appearances of canine and feline GI inflammation and neoplasia can overlap, with changes typically more dramatic and severe with neoplasia and milder and more subtle with inflammation.[3,4,14] In many cases of gastritis and enteritis, no ultrasound changes are visible. However, findings consistent with GI inflammation include diffuse or multifocal mild wall thickening, loss of definition of wall layers, and mesenteric lymphadenopathy (**Fig. 13**).[3,4,14–16] In one study, dogs with enteritis had an average wall thickness of 0.6 cm. In separate studies, however, small intestinal wall thickening was not sensitive or specific for enteritis, and normal bowel wall thickness should not rule out inflammatory disease.[15,17] Bowel wall layering can appear normal in the face of inflammation but may also have a mild loss of definition. Increased prominence of the muscularis layer (equal or greater in thickness to the

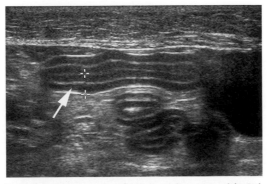

Fig. 15. Longitudinal image of a segment of jejunum in a cat with GI lymphosarcoma. The muscularis layer (*arrow*) is prominent and thickened, and overall bowel wall thickening is present (measured between calipers). Note the similarity in appearance to inflammatory bowel disease in **Fig. 14**.

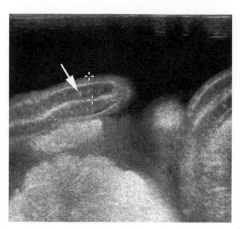

Fig. 16. Longitudinal image of a segment of jejunum in a dog with lymphangiectasia. Anechoic free fluid is present. The mucosal layer contains multiple hyperechoic striations (*arrow*) consistent with dilated lacteals.

mucosal layer) has been reported with inflammatory bowel disease, primarily in the cat (**Fig. 14**).[16,18,19] Chronic partial obstruction can result in hypertrophy of the muscularis layer, giving the same appearance. Intestinal lymphosarcoma can also result in thickening of the muscularis layer and should always be considered as a differential diagnosis for a thickened muscularis layer (**Fig. 15**). Other ultrasound findings associated with enteritis in the dog and cat include mesenteric lymphadenopathy, although lymph node enlargement is usually mild compared with lymph nodes with neoplastic involvement (1.0 cm or less in thickness; normal is ≤5 mm).[14] Hyperechoic speckles and striations within the mucosal layer likely represent dilated lacteals and can be seen with inflammatory bowel disease and lymphangiectasia in the dog (**Fig. 16**).[3,20] Peritoneal effusion frequently accompanies lymphangiectasia. Bowel corrugation or "rippling" (seen best in the submucosal layer) can also occur with enteritis but is a somewhat nonspecific sign (see **Fig. 12**).[21] Corrugation has also been reported with peritonitis, pancreatitis, uroabdomen, bowel ischemia, and lymphosarcoma.

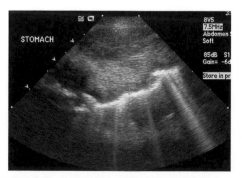

Fig. 17. Longitudinal image of the stomach in a dog with gastric carcinoma. The near wall of the stomach (*between calipers*) is markedly thickened. Alternating hyperechoic and hypoechoic layers are present consistent with pseudolayering. These pseudolayers do not correspond to the normal histopathologic wall layers.

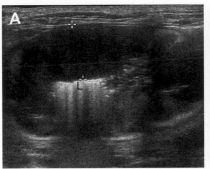
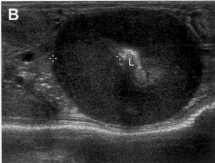

Fig. 18. Transverse images of the stomach (*A*) and duodenum (*B*) in a dog with GI lymphosarcoma. In both stomach and duodenum, the walls are hypoechoic and severely thickened (*between calipers*), with complete loss of layers. The lumen (L) is present as a hyperechoic interface in the center of the stomach and duodenum.

NEOPLASIA

Gastric and intestinal neoplasia most commonly results in more dramatic wall thickening with complete loss of wall layers.[3,4,10,14,22] In one report, the average intestinal wall thickness in dogs with intestinal neoplasia was 1.5 cm, much higher than that reported for enteritis.[14] Complete loss of visualization of wall layering is common with either gastric or intestinal neoplasia and is considered the most specific ultrasound indication of neoplastic disease.[14] Individual wall layers are replaced by a more uniform hypoechoic thickening in many cases, although more complex masses may also occur. Neoplastic masses in the intestines are usually focal, or multifocal, and can be annular or eccentric, extending out of the lumen. Enteritis typically has more diffuse involvement. It should be remembered, however, that some neoplastic lesions are subtle, and difficult to differentiate from inflammation. Mesenteric lymph nodes are usually more dramatically enlarged with neoplastic involvement, with an average thickness of 1.9 cm in one study.[14] Although cytology or histopathology is necessary for a definite diagnosis, some GI tumors have ultrasound characteristics that may allow a preliminary diagnosis. Gastric adenocarcinoma has been reported to cause

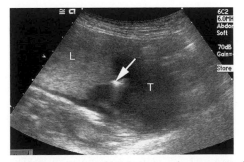

Fig. 19. Longitudinal image of a segment of jejunum in a dog presented for chronic vomiting and weight loss. The lumen (*arrow*) is almost completely obliterated by an intestinal mass (T) growing circumferentially around the jejunum. The portion of bowel orad to the mass (L) is dilated with echogenic fluid secondary to obstruction. The mass was removed surgically and diagnosed as adenocarcinoma.

"pseudolayering," with alternating hypoechoic and hyperechoic layers in the thickened wall that do not correspond to actual histologic wall anatomy (**Fig. 17**).[23] Lymphosarcoma tends to be multifocal or involve long segments of bowel, whereas intestinal adenocarcinoma is more often focal, often causing partial or complete obstruction (**Figs. 18** and **19**).[14,24–27] Leiomyosarcoma originates intramurally and may bulge out of the serosa as an extraluminal mass. The masses often contain hypo/anechoic areas, likely representing central necrosis.[28]

GI inflammatory diseases are best diagnosed with biopsies taken during endoscopy or laparotomy. However, neoplastic masses may be successfully diagnosed using ultrasound-guided, fine-needle aspiration or even tru-cut biopsy if large enough. The bowel or gastric lumen should be avoided during biopsy procedures.

SUMMARY

Ultrasound of the stomach, small bowel, and colon is extremely helpful in the diagnosis of obstructive lesions, inflammation, and neoplastic disease. Although gas can preclude complete visualization of portions of the GI tract, disease processes can often be well visualized. Evaluation of the stomach and bowel should be included in the complete ultrasound examination.

REFERENCES

1. Penninck DG, Nyland TG, Fisher PE, et al. Ultrasonography of the normal canine gastrointestinal tract. Vet Radiol Ultrasound 1989;30:272–6.
2. Newell SM, Graham JP, Roberts GD, et al. Sonography of the normal feline gastrointestinal tract. Vet Radiol Ultrasound 1999;40:40–3.
3. Penninck DG. Gastrointestinal tract. In: Penninck D, D'Anjou MA, editors. Atlas of small animal ultrasonography. Ames (IA): Blackwell Publishing; 2008. p. 281–318.
4. Penninck DG. Gastrointestinal tract. In: Nyland T, Mattoon J, editors. Small animal diagnostic ultrasound. 2nd edition. Philadelphia: WB Saunders; 2002. p. 207–30.
5. Delaney F, O'Brien RT, Waller K. Ultrasound evaluation of small bowel thickness compared to weight in normal dogs. Vet Radiol Ultrasound 2003;44:577–80.
6. Goggin JM, Biller DS, Debey BM, et al. Ultrasonographic measurement of gastrointestinal wall thickness and the ultrasonographic appearance of the ileocolic region in healthy cats. J Am Anim Hosp Assoc 2000;36:224–8.
7. Lamb CR, Forster-van Hijfte M. Beware the gastric pseudomass. Vet Radiol Ultrasound 1994;35:398–9.
8. Tyrell D, Beck C. Survey of the use of radiography vs. ultrasonography in the investigation of gastrointestinal foreign bodies in small animals. Vet Radiol Ultrasound 2006;47:404–8.
9. Tidwell AS, Penninck DG. Ultrasonography of gastrointestinal foreign bodies. Vet Radiol Ultrasound 1992;33:160–9.
10. Penninck DG, Nyland TG, Kerr LY, et al. Ultrasonographic evaluation of gastrointestinal diseases in small animals. Vet Radiol Ultrasound 1990;31:134–41.
11. Lamb CR, Mantis P. Ultrasonographic features of intestinal intussusception in 10 dogs. J Small Anim Pract 1998;39:437–41.
12. Patsikas MN, Papazoglou LG, Papaioannou NG, et al. Ultrasonographic findings of intestinal intussusception in seven cats. J Feline Med Surg 2003;5:335–43.
13. Patsikas MN, Jakovljevic S, Moustardas, et al. Ultrasonographic signs of intestinal intussusception associated with acute enteritis or gastroenteritis in 19 young dogs. J Am Anim Hosp Assoc 2003;39:57–66.

14. Penninck D, Smyers B, Webster C, et al. Diagnostic value of ultrasonography in differentiating enteritis from intestinal neoplasia in dogs. Vet Radiol Ultrasound 2003;44:570–5.
15. Gaschen L, Kircher P, Stüssi A, et al. Comparison of ultrasonographic findings with Clinical Activity Index (CIBDAI) and diagnosis in dogs with chronic enteropathies. Vet Radiol Ultrasound 2008;49:56–64.
16. Baez JL, Hendrick MJ, Walker LM, et al. Radiographic, ultrasonographic, and endoscopic findings in cats with inflammatory bowel disease of the stomach and small intestine: 33 cases (1990–1997). J Am Vet Med Assoc 1999;215: 349–54.
17. Rudorf H, van Schaik G, O'Brien RT, et al. Ultrasonographic evaluation of the thickness of the small intestinal wall in dogs with inflammatory bowel disease. J Small Anim Pract 2005;46:322–6.
18. Bettini G, Muracchini M, Della Salda L, et al. Hypertrophy of intestinal smooth muscle in cats. Res Vet Sci 2003;75:43–53.
19. Diana A, Pietra M, Gugliemini C, et al. Ultrasonographic and pathologic features of intestinal smooth muscle hypertrophy in four cats. Vet Radiol Ultrasound 2003; 44:566–99.
20. Sutherland-Smith J, Penninck DG, Keating JH, et al. Ultrasonographic intestinal hyperechoic mucosal striations in dogs are associated with lacteal dilation. Vet Radiol Ultrasound 2007;48:51–7.
21. Moon ML, Biller DS, Armbrust LJ. Ultrasonographic appearance and etiology of corrugated small intestine. Vet Radiol Ultrasound 2003;44:199–203.
22. Kaser-Hotz B, Hauser B, Arnold P. Ultrasonographic findings in canine gastric neoplasia in 13 patients. Vet Radiol Ultrasound 1996;37:51–6.
23. Penninck DG, Moore AS, Gliatto J. Ultrasonography of canine gastric epithelial neoplasia. Vet Radiol Ultrasound 1998;39:342 8.
24. Penninck DG, Moore AS, Tidwell AS, et al. Ultrasonography of alimentary lymphosarcoma in the cat. Vet Radiol Ultrasound 1994;35:299–304.
25. Grooters AM, Biller DS, Ward H, et al. Ultrasonographic appearance of feline alimentary lymphoma. Vet Radiol Ultrasound 1994;35:468–72.
26. Rivers BJ, Walter PA, Feeney D, et al. Ultrasonographic features of intestinal adenocarcinoma in five cats. Vet Radiol Ultrasound 1997;38:300–6.
27. Paoloni MC, Penninck DG, Moore AS. Ultrasonographic and clinicopathologic findings in 21 dogs with intestinal adenocarcinoma. Vet Radiol Ultrasound 2002;43:562–7.
28. Myers NC, Penninck DG. Ultrasonographic diagnosis of gastrointestinal smooth muscle tumors in the dog. Vet Radiol Ultrasound 1994;35:391–7.

Ultrasound of the Right Lateral Intercostal Space

Erin L. Brinkman-Ferguson, DVM[a],*, David S. Biller, DVM[b]

KEYWORDS
- Ultrasound • Liver • Porta hepatis • Pancreas
- Kidney • Adrenal

Ultrasound is a widely used, safe, noninvasive diagnostic tool in veterinary medicine. Over time, ultrasound equipment has become more sophisticated, yet more afford-able, for many practitioners. However, the quality of an ultrasonographic examination depends on the skill and experience of the individual performing the study. Many sonographers perform an entire abdominal examination from a ventral approach, confining the scan to a subcostal window. Although a subcostal approach may be adequate for some dogs, it may be inadequate for evaluation of the structures of the right cranial abdomen in others. These structures include the right side of the liver, porta hepatis (caudal vena cava, portal vein, and common bile duct), right limb and body of the pancreas, duodenum, right kidney, right adrenal gland, and hepatic lymph nodes. These structures are especially difficult to evaluate via a ventral approach in dogs that are large, deep-chested, have microhepatica, have a large amount of gastrointestinal gas, or have a large volume of peritoneal effusion. For the instances described here, a right lateral intercostal approach is indicated.[1] The technique of the right lateral intercostal approach, normal ultrasonographic anatomy, and clinical indications of this approach are described.

TECHNIQUE AND NORMAL ANATOMY

Very little patient preparation is required for the right lateral intercostal approach. This technique may be easily performed during a standard examination. As with any abdominal ultrasound study, the hair should be adequately clipped. The hair should be clipped dorsally to the level of the epaxial muscles, caudally to the pelvis, and

[a] Department of Clinical Sciences, College of Veterinary Medicine, Mississippi State University, Box 6100, Mississippi State, MS 39762, USA
[b] Department of Clinical Sciences, Kansas State University, Veterinary Medical Teaching Hospital, 1800 Denison Avenue, Manhattan, KS 66506, USA
* Corresponding author.
E-mail address: brinkman@cvm.msstate.edu (E.L. Brinkman-Ferguson).

Vet Clin Small Anim 39 (2009) 761–781
doi:10.1016/j.cvsm.2009.04.007
0195-5616/09/$ – see front matter © 2009 Elsevier Inc. All rights reserved.

vetsmall.theclinics.com

cranially to the region of the diaphragm, which corresponds to approximately the eighth or ninth intercostal space (**Fig. 1**A, B).[2] The animal may be positioned in dorsal or left lateral recumbency. A transducer with a small footprint, or contact surface, should be used to avoid shadowing artifacts from the ribs (see **Fig. 1**B).[1,3] To find the appropriate window, the transducer should first be placed parallel to the ribs from the ninth through twelfth intercostal spaces to achieve an image in the transverse plane. If reverberation artifact is seen due to aerated lung, the transducer should be angled caudally or moved one intercostal space caudally. Long axis images in the dorsal plane can be acquired by turning the transducer 90°, with the left side of the image representing the cranial direction.[1]

Examination of the liver in dogs is more difficult than in people because of its more cranial and upright position under the rib cage. Gastrointestinal gas creates difficulty when scanning from a ventral approach.[4] In most cats and small dogs, the liver can be scanned from behind the ribs. In large and/or deep-chested dogs, this window may be inadequate for examination of the liver. In these cases, the transducer should be placed in the last three to four intercostal spaces for complete evaluation. However, if the liver is decreased in size, the sonographer may still encounter aerated lung when using this approach.[5]

The right lateral intercostal scan plane is indicated for examination of the porta hepatis.[2,4–7] Structures evaluated at the region of the porta hepatis include the aorta, caudal vena cava, portal vein, and common bile duct. There is a narrow acoustic window for examination of these structures through the liver, between the aerated lung and gastrointestinal gas in the right cranial abdomen.[4] To find the porta hepatis, the transducer is placed in a transverse position (dorsal is to the left of the image) at the tenth through twelfth intercostal spaces, approximately 5 to 10 cm ventral to the spine.[1,6] The appropriate window is seen when there is no artifact from air in the lung or gas in the gastrointestinal tract, and the aorta, caudal vena cava, and portal vein are seen. If aerated lung is encountered, the transducer is angled caudally or moved caudally one intercostal space. If the right kidney is seen, the transducer is angled cranially or moved cranially one intercostal space.[1,7] If gas from the gastrointestinal tract is seen, the transducer is moved dorsally and angled ventromedially.[7] The vessels of the porta hepatis are easily distinguished because of their anatomy and spectral Doppler characteristics.[6]

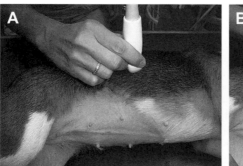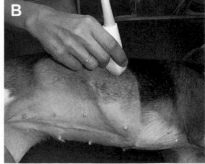

Fig. 1. (*A*) A dog that has been inadequately clipped for a right intercostal approach. Notice the clipped area is confined caudal to the rib cage. (*B*) This dog is adequately prepared for a right intercostal approach. The clipped area extends cranially beyond the costal arch. Note the small size of the transducer's footprint.

The aorta is the most dorsal structure in the region of the porta hepatis and is found on the midline. This vessel demonstrates pulsatility and seems to pass over the diaphragm.[5-7] The diaphragmatic line is seen ventral to the aorta, because the aorta does not go through it but passes dorsal to it (**Figs. 2A–C and 3**).[2]

The caudal vena cava is ventral and slightly to the right of the aorta.[5,6] The caudal vena cava is surrounded by the caudate and right lateral liver lobes as it passes through the liver (see **Fig. 2A–C**).[2] Deep abdominal compression may allow narrowing of this vessel. This is not possible with the aorta.[5] The caudal vena cava demonstrates mild to moderate pulsatility with increased flow during diastole.[6]

The portal vein is ventral and slightly to the left of the caudal vena cava.[5,6,8] The cross-sectional areas of the three vessels is roughly equal (see Figs. 2A–C and 3).[7] The walls of the portal vein are echogenic due to the presence of fat and fibrous tissue.[5,8] Portal vein blood flow is uniform and nonpulsatile.[6,9] On pulsed-wave Doppler, the portal vein demonstrates a wide range of velocities across the lumen (spectral broadening).[6] The mean velocity of portal blood flow is 15 cm/s (12–17 cm/s), with minimal fluctuation over time.[9,10] In normal dogs, the cross-sectional area of the portal vein is slightly greater on expiration than on inspiration.[11] Factors that influence normal portal flow include eating (increase), exercise (decrease), and upright posture (decrease).[10]

The common bile duct is ventral and slightly to the right of the portal vein (**Fig. 4**).[4,5] The common bile duct leaves the liver and enters the duodenum at the major duodenal papilla. The normal common bile duct in dogs measures approximately 1 to 3 mm on ultrasound.[5] The cystic duct, hepatic ducts, and peripheral intrahepatic bile ducts are not seen in normal animals.[4,5] It is difficult to demarcate the end of the cystic duct and the beginning of the common bile duct. However, this demarcation is not necessary in normal dogs.[5]

The hepatic veins are also easily evaluated from the right intercostal approach.[2,8,12] Two hepatic veins enter the caudal vena cava from the right, and one enters from the left.[2] Unlike the portal veins, the walls of the hepatic veins are not echogenic. In a study of 16 normal dogs of various conformations, the best positions for locating and evaluating the caudate and right lateral hepatic veins were from the right ninth through eleventh intercostal spaces half way along the ribs and cranial to the right kidney, with the dogs in left lateral recumbency. The quadrate and right medial hepatic veins were also evaluated from the right. In some dogs in the study, all of the hepatic veins could be seen with the transducer at the costochondral junction at the right seventh or eighth intercostal spaces and angled dorsocranially.[8]

Evaluation of the hepatic veins with two-dimensional imaging and spectral Doppler may be useful in the examination of dogs with heart disease, liver disease, or fluid overload. Doppler interrogation of the hepatic veins may be performed from the right ninth through eleventh intercostal spaces (**Fig. 5A, B**). The right medial and quadrate hepatic veins are easily identified due to their relationship with the gall bladder. Doppler interrogation is most accurate with the vessels imaged in long axis, as close to parallel with the Doppler signal as possible. The movement of blood across the hepatic veins depends on the pressure gradient between the venous pressure in the abdomen and the pressure in the right atrium.[13] On pulsed-wave Doppler, the hepatic veins demonstrate a periodic signal, corresponding to right atrial pressure (**Fig. 6**). The pressure changes in the thorax and abdomen that occur with respiration influence the Doppler waveform. There is increased velocity in the forward direction with inspiration.[12] Doppler interrogation of the hepatic veins may be useful in the evaluation of cardiac disease, hepatic disease, and in dogs with volume overload.[13]

The common hepatic artery is a small structure that is often not seen in normal dogs. It may sometimes be located using a right lateral intercostal approach. The common hepatic artery is a major branch of the celiac artery. It may be found by using a right intercostal approach to locate the first large branch of the celiac artery that courses

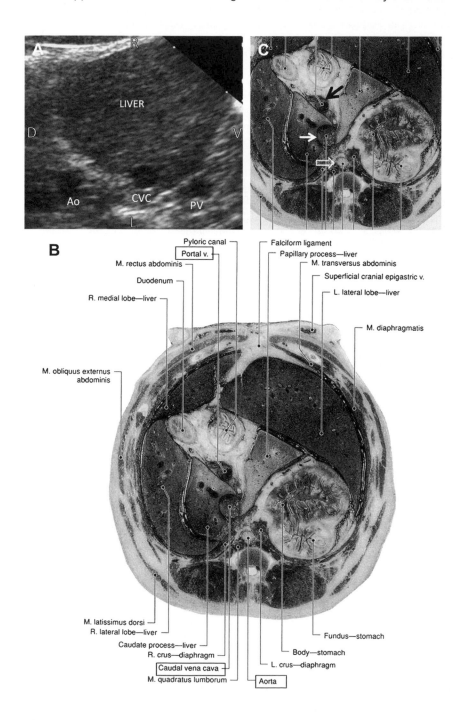

to the porta hepatis (**Fig. 7**). The celiac artery is easily identified because of its close association with the cranial mesenteric artery. The common hepatic artery was interrogated with pulsed-wave Doppler in 10 normal adult beagles, 20 normal puppies, and 7 dogs with hepatic disease. In the normal adult beagles, mean peak systolic velocity was 1.5 m/s (1.1–2.3 m/s), with a resistive index of 0.68 (0.62–0.74). In the normal puppies, the mean peak systolic velocity was lower at 1.0 m/s (0.8–1.3 m/s) with a lower resistive index of 0.59 (0.46–0.65). There were no differences in values obtained after fasting and postprandially. Two dogs with congenital arterioportal fistulae demonstrated higher peak systolic velocity and lower mean resistive index than normal puppies. There were no differences in the normal adult beagles and the five adult dogs with acquired hepatoportal disease.[14] Intrahepatic arteries are not seen in normal animals.[5]

In the past, the normal pancreas was difficult, if not impossible, to evaluate with ultrasound. With improvements in equipment, the normal pancreas is not the elusive structure it once was. However, proper technique is required to image this organ. Complete evaluation is often impossible from a subcostal approach. The right limb and body may be examined with a right lateral intercostal approach. This approach is especially helpful in deep-chested dogs and dogs with pain in the right cranial abdomen.[3] The pancreas consists of a left lobe, body, and right lobe. If seen, the left lobe is typically imaged from a subcostal approach, whereas the body and right limb often require a right intercostal approach (**Fig. 8A–E**). Several structures serve as landmarks for the pancreas. The pancreatic body unites the right and left lobes and can be found caudal to the pylorus, ventral to the portal vein, and craniomedial to the right kidney and caudate process of the caudate lobe of the liver. The right lobe lies in the mesoduodenum, dorsal or dorsomedial to the descending duodenum, ventral to the right kidney, and ventrolateral to the portal vein.[3,15] To make sure that the entire right lobe has been imaged, the descending duodenum should be followed caudally to its caudal flexure.[3] The normal pancreas is isoechoic or slightly hyperechoic to the liver.[3,15]

The only visible veins in the pancreas are those that drain the right lobe. The cranial and caudal parts of the pancreaticoduodenal vein lie in the right lobe and run parallel to the descending duodenum. The descending duodenum is identified by its straight course and prominent walls.[3] The cranial pancreaticoduodenal vein becomes the gastroduodenal vein, which drains into the portal vein near the porta hepatis.[3,16] The caudal pancreaticoduodenal vein meets with the cranial mesenteric vein.[3]

The right kidney is often more difficult than the left to evaluate from a ventral or subcostal approach because of its dorsocranial position in the renal fossa of the caudate lobe of the liver and because it is dorsal to the duodenum and proximal portion of the

---

Fig. 2. (*A*) Transverse right lateral intercostal ultrasonographic image of the porta hepatis in a normal dog. The aorta (Ao) is the most dorsal of the three vascular structures. The caudal vena cava (CVC) is ventral and slightly to the right of the aorta. The portal vein (PV) is ventral and slightly to the left of the caudal vena cava. D, dorsal; R, right; V, ventral; L, left. (*B*) Cross section of a canine cadaver at the level of the twelfth thoracic vertebra. Note the location of the portal vein, caudal vena cava, and aorta. (*Adapted from* Feeney DA, Fletcher TF, Hardy RM. Atlas of correlative imaging anatomy of the normal dog: ultrasound and computed tomography. Philadelphia: WB Saunders; 1991. p. 246; with permission.) (*C*) Same image as **Fig. 3B** magnified to demonstrate the three major blood vessels of the porta hepatis. The portal vein (*black arrow*), caudal vena cava (*solid white arrow*), and aorta (*open white arrow*) are identified. (*Adapted from* Feeney DA, Fletcher TF, Hardy RM. Atlas of correlative imaging anatomy of the normal dog: ultrasound and computed tomography. Philadelphia: WB Saunders; 1991. p. 246; with permission.)

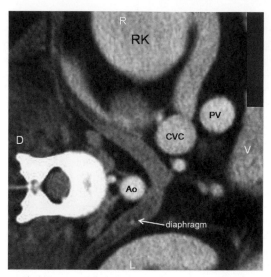

Fig. 3. Transverse image of the cranial abdomen of a dog obtained with computed tomography (CT). Vascular structures are enhanced due to the administration of intravenous iodinated contrast. Note the aorta (Ao) dorsal to the diaphragm. The caudal vena cava (CVC) is ventral and to the right of the aorta. The portal vein (PV) is ventral to the caudal vena cava. RK, right kidney; D, dorsal; R, right; V, ventral; L, left.

colon.[1,17] This is especially true in deep-chested dogs. In these animals, the right kidney should be examined with the transducer placed at the right tenth through twelfth intercostal spaces.[17,18] With the right lateral intercostal approach, the right kidney may be located by moving caudally from the porta hepatis.[1]

The echogenicity of the kidneys relative to the other abdominal organs is evaluated in every thorough abdominal ultrasound examination. Because of its position in the right cranial abdomen, the echogenicity of the right kidney is easily compared to that of the caudate lobe of the liver.[17,19] In normal dogs, the renal cortex is hypoechoic or isoechoic to the liver. The renal cortex is sharply marginated against and is more echogenic than the medulla because of the presence of glomeruli, tubules, and other structures.[17,18,20] The renal diverticula and interlobar vessels are seen as hyperechoic,

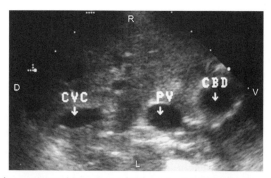

Fig. 4. Transverse ultrasonographic image of the porta hepatis of a dog with severe hepatic disease and biliary obstruction. The common bile duct (CBD) is prominent and lies ventral to the portal vein (PV). D, dorsal; R, right; V, ventral; L, left; CVC, caudal vena cava.

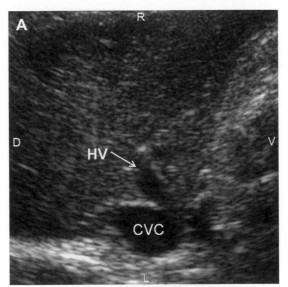

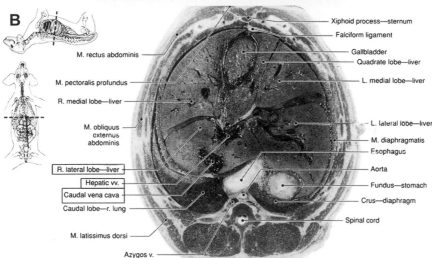

Fig. 5. (*A*) Transverse ultrasound image of the porta hepatis of a normal dog. A hepatic vein (HV) is seen entering the caudal vena cava (CVC). D, dorsal; R, right; V, ventral; L, left. (*B*) Cross-section of a canine cadaver at the level of the tenth thoracic vertebra. Note the relative locations of the caudal vena cava and the right lateral liver lobe and corresponding hepatic vein. (*Adapted from* Feeney DA, Fletcher TF, Hardy RM. Atlas of correlative imaging anatomy of the normal dog: ultrasound and computed tomography. Philadelphia: WB Saunders; 1991. p. 242; with permission.)

linear structures in the medulla.[17] Assuming that the surrounding organs are normal, changes in renal echogenicity may indicate renal disease.[19]

Although small, examination of the adrenal glands is essential for a complete abdominal ultrasound exam. The right adrenal gland is typically more difficult to evaluate than the left, because it is in a more cranial position, creating the need for intercostal imaging in many dogs.[18,21–23] This gland is also difficult to evaluate due to the presence of gas in

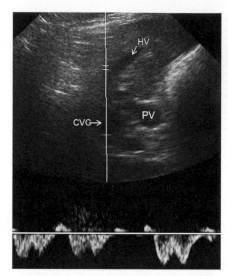

Fig. 6. Duplex-Doppler interrogation of a hepatic vein (HV). Note the normal periodic signal generated within the hepatic vein. The irregular signal above the baseline is an artifact caused by respiratory motion. CVC, caudal vena cava; PV, portal vein.

the pylorus and duodenum, which tends to be more of a problem on the right than on the left.[21] The intercostal approach to the right adrenal gland is especially helpful in large dogs.[2] The celiac and cranial mesenteric arteries, cranial pole of the right kidney, and the caudal vena cava serve as landmarks for locating the right adrenal gland.[1,2,22] The cranial pole of the right kidney is located at the eleventh or twelfth intercostal space and the transducer angled medially. If the caudal vena cava is encountered, the transducer is then angled slightly laterally.[21,22] The right adrenal gland is located at the level of or just cranial to the celiac and cranial mesenteric arteries, between the cranial pole of the right kidney and caudal vena cava (**Fig. 9A–C**).[2,23] In long axis from this window, the right adrenal gland is oval or comma shaped.[21]

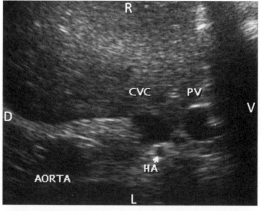

Fig. 7. Right intercostal transverse image at the porta hepatis in a dog. The small hepatic artery (HA) is seen to the left of the caudal vena cava (CVC). D, dorsal; R, right; V, ventral; L, left; PV, portal vein.

Although typically not seen in a normal dog, multiple lymph nodes may be examined via a right intercostal approach.[1] Normal lymph nodes are usually isoechoic to surrounding tissues. Blood vessels or other organs are used as landmarks for locating lymph nodes on ultrasound. The hepatic lymph nodes lie on both sides of the portal vein, approximately 1 to 2 cm caudal to the porta hepatis (**Fig. 10**). The right nodes vary in number from one to five, are adjacent to the body of the pancreas, and are smaller than those on the left. The left is larger at 1 to 6 cm in length and is found in the lesser omentum dorsal to the common bile duct. The hepatic lymph nodes drain the stomach, duodenum, pancreas, and liver. The gastric lymph nodes are inconsistently found in the lesser omentum near the pylorus and right gastric artery and drain the stomach, esophagus, diaphragm, liver, mediastinum, and peritoneum. The pancreaticoduodenal lymph nodes are also inconsistent and may be found in the mesoduodenum and greater omentum. They drain the duodenum, pylorus, and right limb of the pancreas. The lymph nodes described here are part of the celiac lymphocenter of the visceral abdominal lymph nodes.[24]

CLINICAL INDICATIONS

The right lateral intercostal ultrasound scan plane is indicated in some dogs for evaluation of diseases involving the right lateral, right medial, and caudate lobes of the liver, especially in large and deep-chested dogs and in cases of microhepatica or large volumes of peritoneal effusion. In large or deep-chested dogs, mass or nodular lesions of the right aspect of the liver may be missed if only a subcostal approach is used (**Fig. 11**).[1] If mass lesions are detected in other abdominal organs, it is important to thoroughly examine the liver. The liver is commonly the first organ where metastasis is seen, because many abdominal organs are drained by the portal vein.[25]

When the liver is small, there may be a very small window of visible hepatic tissue between the aerated lung and gas in the stomach.[5] Conditions that may cause microhepatica include cirrhosis, congenital portosystemic shunts, or other chronic diseases of the liver.[1]

The "classic" combination of ultrasonographic findings in hepatic cirrhosis includes a small, irregularly marginated, hyperechoic liver with nodules and peritoneal effusion. However, in a study of 55 dogs and two cats with a histopathologic diagnosis of hepatic cirrhosis, this classic appearance was seen only in 5% of the cases. Four dogs (7%) had a normal study. The most common finding in this study was peritoneal effusion in 62%, followed by irregular liver margination in 53%, and hepatic nodules in 51%. More livers were normal in size (55%) and echogenicity (51%) than were small (34%) and hyperechoic (38%).[26] The "classic" form of cirrhosis may be detected only late in the disease process.[27] However, the right lateral intercostal view is still indicated due to the presence of effusion.

Cirrhosis is the most common cause of portal hypertension in dogs.[27] In a study of 10 normal dogs and 10 dogs with surgically induced hepatic cirrhosis, the portal vein was interrogated with pulsed-wave Doppler. The transducer was placed at the right eleventh or twelfth intercostal space for these examinations. Mean portal flow and mean portal flow velocity were decreased in dogs with cirrhosis. The portal vein diameter was unchanged.[11]

Congenital portosystemic shunts are abnormal vascular connections between the portal venous system and the systemic venous system. Most congenital, single extrahepatic portosystemic shunts connect a major tributary of the portal vein and the caudal vena cava, cranial to the phrenicoabdominal veins. In dogs, the shunt vessel usually arises from the main portal vein, splenic vein, or left gastric vein.[16] These

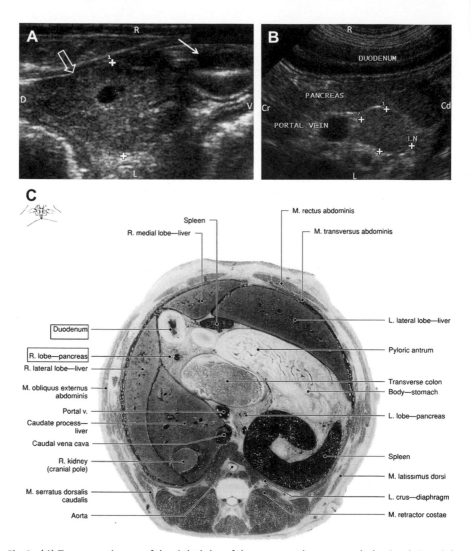

Fig. 8. (*A*) Transverse image of the right lobe of the pancreas (*open arrow*) obtained via a right lateral intercostal approach in a dog. The duodenum (*solid white arrow*) is ventral to the pancreas. D, dorsal; R, right; V, ventral; L, left. (*B*) Long axis right intercostal view of the right lobe of the pancreas in a dog with lymphoma. The pancreas is ventrolateral to the portal vein (PV). An enlarged hepatic lymph node (LN) is present medial to the pancreas. Cr, cranial; R, right; Cd, caudal; L, left. (*C*) Cross section of a canine cadaver at the level of T13-L1. Note the relative locations of the duodenum and right lobe of the pancreas. (*Adapted from* Feeney DA, Fletcher TF, Hardy RM. Atlas of correlative imaging anatomy of the normal dog: ultrasound and computed tomography. Philadelphia: WB Saunders; 1991. p. 248; with permission.) (*D*) Cross section of a canine cadaver at the level of the third lumbar vertebra. Note the location of the right lobe of the pancreas and its association with the descending duodenum and right kidney. (*Adapted from* Feeney DA, Fletcher TF, Hardy RM. Atlas of correlative imaging anatomy of the normal dog: ultrasound and computed tomography. Philadelphia: WB Saunders; 1991. p. 254; with permission.) (*E*) Same image as that in Fig. 9D, magnified to demonstrate the positions of the right lobe of the pancreas (*arrow*), descending duodenum (D), and right kidney (RK). (*Adapted from* Feeney DA, Fletcher TF, Hardy RM. Atlas of correlative imaging anatomy of the normal dog: ultrasound and computed tomography. Philadelphia: WB Saunders; 1991. p. 254; with permission.)

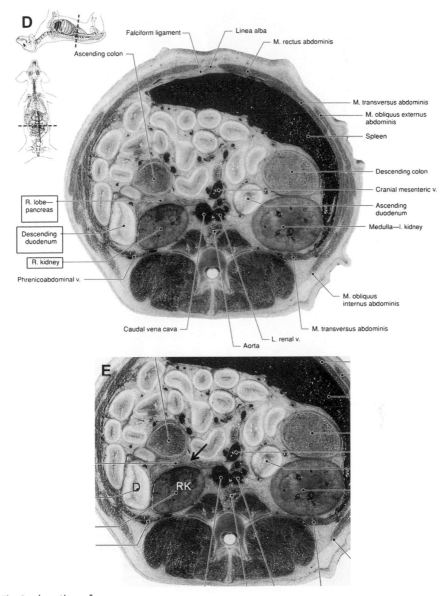

Fig. 8. (*continued*)

anomalous vessels may present a diagnostic challenge. The right lateral intercostal approach is indicated in any suspected congenital portosystemic shunt.[9,28] In a study of 82 dogs with clinical and/or clinicopathologic signs consistent with portosystemic shunt, the condition was confirmed in 38 via mesenteric portography. Ultrasound was 95% sensitive, 98% specific, and 94% accurate for congenital portosystemic shunts.[9]

Two-dimensional ultrasonographic findings with portosystemic shunts may include microhepatica, decreased visibility of the intrahepatic portal veins, and an abnormal blood vessel draining into the caudal vena cava (**Fig. 12**).[9] It is recommended to

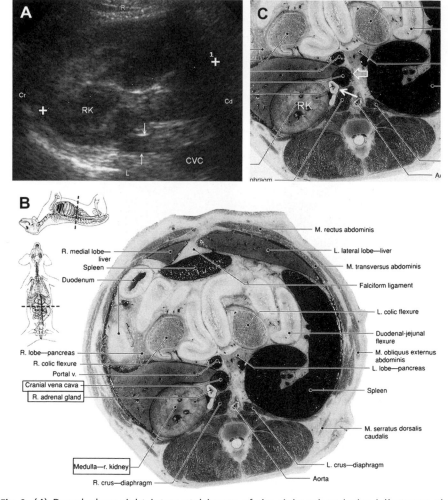

Fig. 9. (*A*) Dorsal plane right intercostal image of the right adrenal gland (*between the arrows*) in a normal dog. The right adrenal gland is located between the cranial pole of the right kidney (RK) and the caudal vena cava (CVC). Cd, caudal; Cr, cranial; L, left R, right. (*B*) Cross section of a canine cadaver at the level of the first lumbar vertebra. Note the relative locations of the right adrenal gland, caudal vena cava, and right kidney. (*Adapted from* Feeney DA, Fletcher TF, Hardy RM. Atlas of correlative imaging anatomy of the normal dog: ultrasound and computed tomography. Philadelphia: WB Saunders; 1991. p. 250; with permission.) (*C*) Same image as in **Fig.10**B, magnified to demonstrate the right adrenal gland (*solid white arrow*), caudal vena cava (*open white arrow*), and right kidney (RK). (*Adapted from* Feeney DA, Fletcher TF, Hardy RM. Atlas of correlative imaging anatomy of the normal dog: ultrasound and computed tomography. Philadelphia: WB Saunders; 1991. p. 246; with permission.)

look for the shunt vessel where it enters the caudal vena cava rather than looking for all of the tributaries of the portal vein (**Fig. 13**).[16]

Portoazygos shunts, in which the shunt vessel communicates with the azygos vein rather than the caudal vena cava, are a less common type of congenital, single, extrahepatic portosystemic shunt. Using the right lateral intercostal window, the shunt

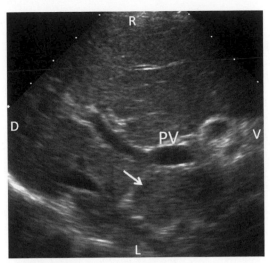

Fig. 10. Right lateral transverse ultrasound image at the porta hepatis in a dog with lymphoma. An enlarged, hypoechoic hepatic lymph node (*arrow*) is seen to the left of the portal vein (PV). D, dorsal; L, left; R, right; V, ventral.

vessel is seen coursing cranial to the diaphragm. It runs parallel to and near the caudal vena cava but does not enter it.[16] The azygos vein is parallel and to the right of the aorta and is rarely seen in normal dogs.[12]

The right lateral intercostal approach is also useful in the evaluation of congenital intrahepatic portosystemic shunts. These anomalous vessels are classified by the division of the liver they affect. Left-divisional intrahepatic shunts are consistent with patent ductus venosus and have a consistent morphology. With this type of shunt, the abnormal vessel courses through the left division and connects the portal vein and caudal vena cava via the left hepatic vein. From a right lateral intercostal approach in a retrospective study of 13 dogs and four cats with a left-divisional shunt, an intrahepatic portal vessel was found to bend to the left and away from the transducer. In the same study, 13 dogs had a central-divisional shunt, which was easy to see from

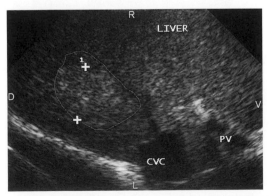

Fig. 11. Transverse intercostal image of the porta hepatis in a dog with an indistinctly margin-ated, hyperechoic nodule (*dashed outline*) in the right aspect of the liver. The nodule was not visible from a subcostal approach. CVC, caudal vena cava; D, dorsal; L, left; PV, portal vein; R, right; V, ventral.

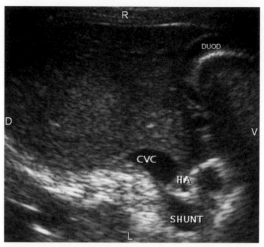

Fig. 12. Right intercostal view of the porta hepatis in a puppy with a single, extrahepatic, portocaval shunt. The shunt vessel is tortuous and is seen entering the caudal vena cava (CVC). D, dorsal; DUOD, duodenum; HA, hepatic artery; L, left; R, right; V, ventral.

the right lateral intercostal view. In those dogs, there was marked aneurysmal dilation of the portal vein. Right-divisional shunts were seen in two dogs and one cat and demonstrated a large, tortuous vessel that coursed far to the right of the midline. Right-divisional and central-divisional shunts had variable morphology, making them difficult to classify on ultrasound.[28]

Several large breeds are predisposed to intrahepatic shunts. Irish wolfhounds are predisposed to left-divisional intrahepatic shunts (patent ductus venosus), whereas

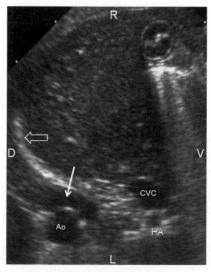

Fig. 13. Dorsal plane intercostal image of the liver of a puppy with a portoazygos shunt (*solid arrow*). The abnormal vessel does not enter the caudal vena cava (CVC) but courses cranial to the diaphragm (*open arrow*) and is seen adjacent to the aorta (Ao). D, dorsal; HA, hepatic artery; L, left; R, right; V, ventral.

Old English sheepdogs are predisposed to central-divisional shunts. Australian cattle dogs are predisposed to right-sided and central-divisional shunts. Retrievers are predisposed to multiple types of intrahepatic shunt morphologies.[28]

Intrahepatic shunts are typically large and easy to find (**Fig. 14**). However, it is important to evaluate their morphology as thoroughly as possible. The type of intrahepatic shunt is an important determinant of whether or not surgical correction is feasible.[28] A left-divisional intrahepatic shunt is consistent with a patent ductus venosus and can be treated by attenuating the left hepatic vein or the shunt vessel where it enters the left hepatic vein. Right-divisional and central-divisional shunts are more difficult to approach surgically.[28]

The use of color and spectral Doppler may increase the sensitivity of ultrasound for the detection of portosystemic shunts.[9,16] Color Doppler may demonstrate turbulent blood flow at the site of entrance of the shunt vessel and may confirm the presence of the abnormal vessel.[9] The normal portal vein has intestinal capillaries at one end and hepatic sinusoids at the other, keeping it unexposed to the pressure variability seen in the arteries and systemic veins.[16] The normal caudal vena cava demonstrates variable pressure and flow because of changing right atrial and pleural pressures throughout the cardiac and respiratory cycles.[9] In dogs with congenital portosystemic shunts, the portal vein is exposed to the same pressure changes as the caudal vena cava, so portal flow may be more variable. Its diameter may change with the cardiac and respiratory cycles like the caudal vena cava. Because these shunts have low resistance to flow, portal flow velocity may also be increased.[9,16] In a prospective study of 38 dogs with confirmed congenital portosystemic shunt, 70% had increased and/or variable portal flow velocity.[9]

In the authors' experience, the common hepatic artery is enlarged and easily seen in some dogs with portosystemic shunts (see **Figs. 12** and **13**). The liver is a highly perfused organ, receiving 25% of cardiac output. Approximately one-third of its blood supply comes from the hepatic artery. Approximately two-thirds comes from the portal vein. Flow from the hepatic artery and portal vein adjust to keep total hepatic flow constant. If one source of flow is decreased, the other increases and vice versa.[14] Increased flow from the hepatic artery may protect the liver in dogs with portosystemic shunts.[14,27]

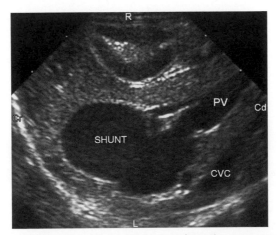

Fig. 14. Right intercostal view of a puppy with an intrahepatic portosystemic shunt. A large tortuous shunt vessel is seen coming from the portal vein (PV). Its termination at the caudal vena cava (CVC) is not visible in this image. Cd, caudal; Cr, cranial; L, left; R, right.

Congenital hepatic arterioportal fistulas may cause portosystemic shunting. This condition may be difficult to diagnose, because it demonstrates features of both congenital and acquired portosystemic shunts on ultrasound.[16] These conditions may all form a complex pattern of dilated vessels in the liver.[29] However, arterioportal fistulas demonstrate reversed, pulsatile portal flow and signs of portal hypertension, such as peritoneal effusion and hepatofugal blood flow.[16,29]

Portal vein thrombosis is an uncommon complication of portosystemic shunt ligation in dogs.[30–32] However, ante mortem diagnosis of spontaneously occurring portal vein thrombosis is rare.[32] Conditions appropriate for the development of thromboemboli include a hypercoagulable state, vascular stasis, and vascular endothelial damage.[33] Reported causes of spontaneous portal vein thrombosis in dogs include ehrlichiosis, pancreatitis, autoimmune disease, renal amyloidosis, sepsis, peritonitis, and retrograde growth of hepatic tumors.[32,33] In many cases, the cause is never determined. Neoplasia can cause portal vein thrombosis by direct invasion into the vessel lumen (tumor thrombus) or by distorting the vessel wall and causing a blood clot.[32]

Portal vein thromboses are best seen using a right lateral intercostal view.[32] Ultrasonographic findings associated with portal vein thrombosis include echogenic material in the venous lumen, peritoneal effusion due to portal hypertension, and dilation of the portal vein (**Fig. 15A, B**).[32,33] If the thrombus is causing complete vessel obstruction, no flow around it will be seen on color Doppler. If the thrombus is not obstructive, there may still be flow around it on color Doppler.[32]

A right intercostal window is often useful for evaluation of disease of the biliary tract, as it is commonly difficult to evaluate from a ventral approach (**Fig. 16A, B**).[4] Extrahepatic biliary obstruction may be caused by neoplasia of the liver, gall bladder, bile ducts, pancreas, gastrointestinal tract, and lymph nodes; cholelithiasis; abscesses; granuloma; or fibrosis due to trauma or inflammation.[4,5] Ultrasound is a useful tool for the detection of extrahepatic biliary obstruction. With obstruction of the common bile duct, the common bile duct becomes enlarged by 24 to 48 hours. The gall bladder reaches its maximum size by 48 hours.[4] Intrahepatic bile duct distention is seen by 5 to 7 days.[4,34] Compared with hepatic veins and intrahepatic portal veins, the intrahepatic bile ducts are more tortuous with irregular borders and do not demonstrate flow on color Doppler. It is not possible to determine the duration of obstruction based on

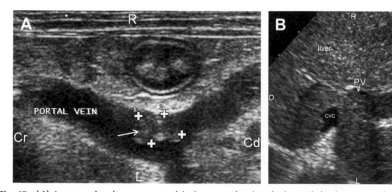

Fig. 15. (*A*) Long-axis ultrasonographic image obtained via a right intercostal approach in a dog with an adrenal tumor and tumor thrombus (*arrow*) in the portal vein. Note the irregularly shaped, echogenic material in the vessel lumen. Cd, caudal; Cr, cranial; L, left; R, right. (*B*) Right intercostal image of the liver of a dog with a thrombus in the portal vein (PV). The normally anechoic lumen of the portal vein is nearly completely obscured by the echogenic thrombus. CVC, caudal vena cava; D, dorsal; L, left; R, right; V, ventral.

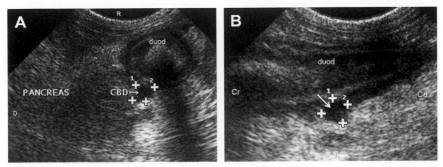

Fig.16. (A) Transverse right intercostal image of the pancreas and common bile duct (CBD) in a dog with pancreatitis and secondary biliary inflammation. The enlarged, hypoechoic pancreas is seen dorsomedial to the duodenum (duod). The mesentery surrounding the pancreas is hyperechoic. D, dorsal; L, left; R, right; V, ventral. (B) Long-axis intercostal image of the same dog in **Fig.17**A. The enlarged common bile duct (*arrow*) is seen near its entrance into the duodenum (duod). Note the undulating duodenum and the surrounding hyperechoic mesentery. Cd, caudal; Cr, cranial; L, left; R, right.

the size of the ducts.[4] The biliary system may remain dilated even after the obstruction has been relieved.[5]

Pancreatic disease, especially pancreatitis, is a common disease in small animals. Ultrasound is an important diagnostic tool for detection of pancreatitis, determining the severity of the disease, identifying involvement of the duodenum, and discovering the presence of other disease complications.[3] Ultrasound is sensitive, safe, noninvasive, and allows the sonographer to differentiate diffuse pancreatic enlargement versus discrete mass lesions.[35] In many animals with pancreatitis, it may be difficult to image the entire organ from a subcostal approach.[1] Reasons for incomplete subcostal evaluation include interference due to gas in the gastrointestinal tract and pain associated with the disease.[3] An intercostal approach may also be less painful, as the sonographer cannot apply much pressure to the region.[1] This approach allows the examiner to avoid bowel gas.[1,15]

Consistent landmarks for the right pancreatic lobe in dogs with pancreatitis include the right kidney and descending duodenum. The vascular landmarks used in normal dogs may not be visible in cases of pancreatitis because of surrounding inflammation and bowel gas. With pancreatitis, the pancreas becomes hypoechoic, and the surrounding mesentery becomes hyperechoic (**Fig. 17**A, B).[15] In some dogs, there may be ill-defined masses that correspond to areas of pancreatic swelling, inflammation, and hemorrhage.[35] There may be free abdominal fluid. The duodenum may be dilated, fluid-filled, atonic, and demonstrate wall thickening. The descending duodenum may also be displaced ventrally and/or laterally.[15] In some dogs with pancreatitis, the right lobe of the pancreas may shift lateral to the duodenum rather than maintaining its normal position medial to the duodenum.[35] Pancreatitis may lead to biliary obstruction and fibrosis with resulting dilation of the common bile duct.[3] Other pancreatic diseases such as neoplasia, cysts, or abscess may be evaluated via the right lateral intercostal approach.[1]

The right lateral intercostal approach may also be useful for evaluation of disease of the right kidney, especially in large and deep-chested dogs and in dogs with gas in the gastrointestinal tract.[1] This window also allows comparison of the relative echogenicities of the liver and right kidney. In normal dogs, the renal cortex is hypoechoic or isoechoic to the liver.[17,18,20] The renal cortex may be hyperechoic relative to the liver in

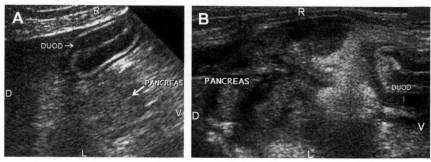

Fig. 17. (A) Transverse intercostal image of the right cranial abdomen of a dog with mild pancreatitis. The pancreas is inhomogeneous and hypoechoic. The mesentery surrounding the pancreas is hyperechoic. (B) Transverse image of the right limb of the pancreas obtained via an intercostal approach in a dog with severe pancreatitis. The pancreas is edematous and severely enlarged and is shifted to a dorsal/dorsolateral position relative to the duodenum (DUOD). The surrounding mesentery is hyperechoic. There is thickening of the duodenal wall. D, dorsal; DUOD, duodenum; L, left; R, right; V, ventral.

conditions such as nephrotoxicosis or nephrocalcinosis (**Fig. 18**).[1] The right intercostal approach may be especially helpful in cases of chronic renal disease in which the kidneys are small or in focal renal disease, such as masses, infarcts, or cysts.[1]

Ultrasound is commonly used to examine the adrenal glands. The right is generally more difficult to evaluate than the left due to its more cranial position and its proximity to the pylorus and duodenum. The right intercostal window is helpful in the detection of diffuse adrenal gland enlargement, such as with pituitary-dependent hyperadreno-corticism, adrenal mass lesions, and invasion or compression of the caudal vena cava by an adrenal lesion (**Fig. 19**A–C).[1,18]

The normal lymph nodes of the right cranial abdomen, such as the hepatic, pancreaticoduodenal, and gastric lymph nodes, are usually not seen in normal animals, because they are small and isoechoic to surrounding tissues.[1,24] When abnormal,

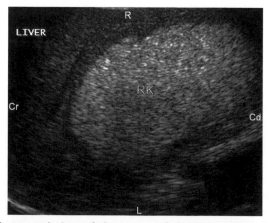

Fig. 18. Long-axis intercostal view of the cortex of the right kidney (RK) in a dog with ethylene glycol toxicity. The right renal cortex is markedly hyperechoic relative to the liver. Cd, caudal; Cr, cranial; L, left; R, right.

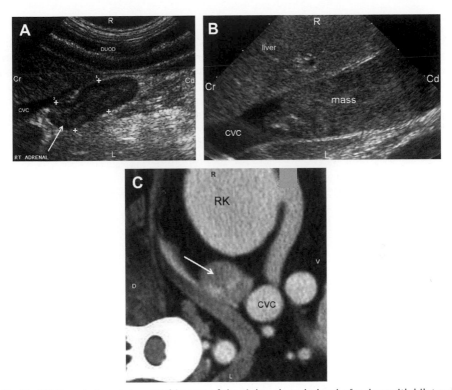

Fig. 19. (*A*) Dorsal plane intercostal image of the right adrenal gland of a dog with bilateral adrenal gland enlargement due to pituitary-dependent hyperadrenocorticism. The adrenal gland is adjacent to the caudal vena cava (CVC), which is being compressed. Cd, caudal; Cr, cranial; DUOD, duodenum; L, left; R, right. (*B*) Long axis intercostal image of a dog with a tumor of the right adrenal gland. The adrenal mass (mass) has invaded the lumen of the caudal vena cava (CVC). Cd, caudal; Cr, cranial; L, left; R, right. (*C*) Transverse computed tomographic image of the cranial abdomen of a dog with a tumor of the right adrenal gland (*arrow*) after intravenous administration of iodinated contrast. The adrenal gland (*arrow*) is enlarged and can be found between the cranial pole of the right kidney (RK) and the caudal vena cava (CVC). D, dorsal; L, left; R, right; V, ventral.

due to neoplasia or inflammation, these lymph nodes may be enlarged and/or hypo-echoic, making them easier to detect.[24]

Cytologic or histopathologic examination of lesions is essential for the diagnosis of many diseases. Ultrasound is a fast, safe, and relatively inexpensive way to locate lesions and obtain samples for microscopic evaluation. Ultrasound is used to view needle placement during fine-needle aspiration or when obtaining a core biopsy, thereby increasing the chance of obtaining a diagnostic sample while avoiding surrounding blood vessels.[36] In a study of 98 dogs and 16 cats, tissue core samples obtained with an 18-gauge biopsy needle were diagnostic in 92% of hepatic biopsies and 100% of renal biopsies.[37] Lesions of the right aspect of the liver or right kidney may be most easily accessed using the right lateral intercostal approach.[1,20] Contra-indications for biopsy include increased bleeding time, decreased platelet count, and increased prothrombin time and partial thromboplastin time. The abdomen should be examined for the presence of hemorrhage following the biopsy procedure and the patient monitored for any signs of bleeding.[20]

SUMMARY

When performing an abdominal ultrasound, a ventral or subcostal approach may be inadequate for a thorough examination. A right lateral intercostal window may be necessary for complete evaluation of the right cranial abdomen. Structures evaluated with this intercostal approach include the right aspect of the liver, porta hepatis, pancreas, proximal duodenum, right kidney, right adrenal gland, and several lymph nodes. Dogs for which this window may be most useful include large and deep-chested dogs, dogs with large volumes of peritoneal effusion or gas in the gastrointestinal tract, and cases of microhepatica and abdominal pain. The right intercostal approach is simple and requires little patient preparation.

REFERENCES

1. Brinkman EL, Biller DS, Armbrust LJ, et al. The clinical utility of the right lateral intercostal scan technique in dogs. J Am Anim Hosp Assoc 2007;43:179–86.
2. Spaulding KA. A review of sonographic identification of abdominal blood vessels and juxtavascular organs. Vet Radiol Ultrasound 1997;38(1):4–23.
3. Saunders HM. Ultrasonography of the pancreas. Probl Vet Med 1991;3(4): 583–603.
4. Nyland TG, Gillett NA. Sonographic evaluation of experimental bile duct ligation in the dog. Vet Radiol 1982;23(6):252–60.
5. Partington BP, Biller DS. Hepatic imaging with radiology and ultrasound. Vet Clin North Am Small Anim Pract 1995;25(2):305–35.
6. Kantrowitz BM, Nyland TG, Fisher P. Estimation of portal blood flow using duplex real-time and pulsed Doppler ultrasound imaging in the dog. Vet Radiol 1989; 30(5):222–6.
7. Szatmári V, Rothizen J, Voorhout G. Standard planes for ultrasonographic examination of the portal system in dogs. J Am Vet Med Assoc 2004;224(5):713–6.
8. Wu JX, Carlisle CH. Ultrasonographic examination of the canine liver based on recognition of hepatic and portal veins. Vet Radiol Ultrasound 1995;36(3):234–9.
9. Lamb CR. Ultrasonographic diagnosis of congenital portosystemic shunts in dogs: results of a prospective study. Vet Radiol Ultrasound 1996;37(4):281–8.
10. Lamb CR, Mahoney PN. Comparison of three methods for calculating portal blood flow velocity in dogs using duplex-Doppler ultrasonography. Vet Radiol Ultrasound 1994;35(3):190–4.
11. Nyland TG, Fisher PE. Evaluation of experimentally induced canine hepatic cirrhosis using duplex Doppler ultrasound. Vet Radiol 1990;31(4):189–94.
12. Szatzmári V, Sótonyi P, Vörös K. Normal duplex Doppler waveforms of major abdominal blood vessels in dogs: a review. Vet Radiol Ultrasound 2001;42(2): 93–107.
13. Smithenson BT, Mattoon JS, Bonagura JD, et al. Pulsed-wave Doppler ultrasonographic evaluation of hepatic veins during variable hemodynamic states in healthy anesthetized dogs. Am J Vet Res 2004;65(6):734–40.
14. Lamb CR, Burton CA, Carlisle CH. Doppler measurement of hepatic arterial flow in dogs: technique and preliminary findings. Vet Radiol Ultrasound 1999;40(1): 77–81.
15. Nyland TG, Mulvany MH, Strombeck DR. Ultrasonic features of experimentally induced, acute pancreatitis in the dog. Vet Radiol 1983;24(6):260–6.
16. Lamb CR. Ultrasonography of portosystemic shunts in dogs and cats. Vet Clin North Am Small Anim Pract 1998;28(4):725–53.

17. Widmer WR, Biller DS, Adams LG. Ultrasonography of the urinary tract in small animals. J Am Vet Med Assoc 2004;225(1):46–54.
18. Lamb CR. Abdominal ultrasonography in small animals: intestinal tract and mesentery, kidneys, adrenal glands, uterus, and prostate. J Small Anim Pract 1990;31:295–304.
19. Hartzband LE, Tidwell AS, Lamb CR. Relative Echogenicity of the renal cortex and liver in normal dogs [abstract]. Br J Radiol 1991;64:654.
20. Smith S. Ultrasound-guided biopsy. Vet Clin North Am Small Anim Pract 1985; 15(6):1249–62.
21. Grooters AM, Biller DS, Miyabayashi T, et al. Evaluation of routine abdominal ultrasonography as a technique for imaging the canine adrenal glands. J Am Anim Hosp Assoc 1994;30:457–62.
22. Tidwell AS, Pennick DG, Besso JG. Imaging of adrenal gland disorders. Vet Clin North Am Small Anim Pract 1997;27(2):237–54.
23. Kantrowitz BM, Nyland TG, Feldman EC. Adrenal ultrasonography in the dog: detection of tumors and hyperplasia in hyperadrenocorticism. Vet Radiol 1986; 27(3):91–6.
24. Pugh CR. Ultrasonographic examination of abdominal lymph nodes in the dog. Vet Radiol Ultrasound 1994;35(2):110–5.
25. Nyman HT, Kristensen AT, Flagstad A, et al. A review of the sonographic assessment of tumor metastasis in liver and superficial lymph nodes. Vet Radiol Ultrasound 2004;45(5):438–48.
26. O'Brien RT. A retrospective study on the sonographic and clinicopathologic features of cirrhosis in dogs and cats [abstract]. Vet Radiol Ultrasound 1999; 40(6):659.
27. Salwei RM, O'Brien RT, Matheson JS. Use of contrast harmonic ultrasound for the diagnosis of congenital portosystemic shunts in three dogs. Vet Radiol Ultrasound 2003;44(3):301–5.
28. Lamb CR, White RN. Morphology of congenital intrahepatic portocaval shunts in dogs and cats. Vet Rec 1998;142:55–60.
29. d'Anjou MA. Huneault L. Imaging Diagnosis—complex intrahepatic portosystemic shunt in a dog. Vet Radiol Ultrasound 2008;49(1):51–5.
30. Mathews K, Gofton N. Congenital extrahepatic portosystemic shunt occlusion in the dog: gross observations during surgical correction. J Am Anim Hosp Assoc 1988;24:387–94.
31. Roy RG, Post GS, Waters DJ, et al. Portal vein thrombosis as a complication of portosystemic shunt ligation in two dogs. J Am Anim Hosp Assoc 1992;28: 53–8.
32. Lamb CR, Wrigley RH, Simpson KW, et al. Ultrasonographic diagnosis of portal vein thrombosis in four dogs. Vet Radiol Ultrasound 1996;37(2):121–9.
33. Bressler C, Himes LC, Moreau RE. Portal vein and aortic thromboses in a Siberian husky with ehrlichiosis and hypothyroidism. J Small Anim Pract 2003;44:408–10.
34. Zeman RK, Taylor KJW, Rosenfield AT, et al. Acute experimental biliary obstruction in the dog: sonographic findings and clinical implications. AJR Am J Roentgenol 1981;136:965–7.
35. Murtaugh RJ, Herring DS, Jacobs RM, et al. Pancreatic ultrasonography in dogs with experimentally induced pancreatitis. Vet Radiol 1985;26(1):27–32.
36. Burkhard MJ, Meyer DJ. Invasive cytology of internal organs: cytology of the thorax and abdomen. Vet Clin North Am Small Anim Pract 1996;26(5):1203–22.
37. Barr F. Percutaneous biopsy of abdominal organs under ultrasound guidance. J Small Anim Pract 1995;36:105–13.

CT Diagnosis of Portosystemic Shunts

Allison Zwingenberger, DVM, MAS

KEYWORDS
- Liver • Shunt • Vascular anomaly • Computed tomography
- Angiography

Portosystemic shunts and other hepatic vascular anomalies are well-known clinical conditions that present a diagnostic challenge. Many are congenital abnormalities and present with typical clinical signs early in an animal's life. Others are the result of alterations in the compliance of hepatic parenchyma and develop in older animals secondary to portal hypertension. This broad group of conditions results in altered hepatic blood supply. Portosystemic shunts have systemic consequences requiring surgical or medical management and often shorten the lifespan of the patient.

Many different modalities in diagnostic imaging can provide information about portosystemic shunts, all with advantages and limitations. Portal angiography involves catheterization of jejunal veins to inject contrast into the portal system for fluoroscopy or radiographs.[1] Nuclear medicine has been used to detect the presence of a shunt by administering radionuclides that are absorbed into the portal vein and quantifying the amount of radionuclide bypassing the liver.[2] More recently, ultrasound has become a diagnostic tool that is capable of visualizing abnormal vasculature directly and evaluating directions of blood flow.[3] Magnetic resonance angiography has also been explored in dogs as a volumetric angiography method.[4] Ultrasound and nuclear scintigraphy are commonly used alone or in combination to diagnose a portosystemic shunt. The essential qualities needed for an imaging modality to diagnose portal vascular anomalies are spatial resolution, contrast resolution, and ability to depict the three-dimensional anatomy of the abdominal vasculature.

Computed tomography is well suited to perform angiography because of fast scan times, good spatial, contrast, and temporal resolution, and the ability to render multiplanar and three-dimensional (3D) images. In the abdomen, where there is a large volume of organs and tissues that surround the vasculature in question, axial images have a clear advantage over two-dimensional planar images. Computed tomographic (CT) angiography is rapidly becoming the gold standard for human vascular imaging and is a new modality for evaluating the hepatic and portal vasculature in animals.[5–10]

Department of Surgical and Radiological Sciences, School of Veterinary Medicine, University of California, Davis, 1 Shields Avenue, 2112 Tupper Hall, Davis, CA 95616, USA
E-mail address: azwingen@ucdavis.edu

Vet Clin Small Anim 39 (2009) 783–792
doi:10.1016/j.cvsm.2009.04.008
0195-5616/09/$ – see front matter © 2009 Published by Elsevier Inc.
vetsmall.theclinics.com

HELICAL CT SCANNING

Technology has advanced extremely quickly since the first CT machine was put into operation in the 1970s. With the advent of helical CT, large volumes of data such as those from the liver could be scanned in a very short period of time. This capability provided the opportunity to use CT for angiography.

Early CT machines used axial scanning techniques that took several minutes to perform. The x-ray tube generated high-energy x-rays to take a 360° image of the body. This information could then be reconstructed into a two-dimensional image or "slice" of the area. After the rotation, the tube current paused, and the table moved the patient into the gantry of the CT by a small increment. The tube then acquired another image, repeating this sequence for the length of the desired acquisition. The average scan was too long to complete before a vascular contrast bolus dissipated.

Helical CT scanning made scan times short enough for angiography. The mechanism of the rotating x-ray tube was altered so that it could rotate continuously instead of pausing to reset. In addition, the table could move constantly at a set rate as the tube was rotating. The result of these modifications was a continuous scan with the data acquired as a volume in a helical fashion. Additional image reconstruction algorithms were also developed to construct axial images from this volume of data. CT machines with multiple parallel detectors are now becoming standard and allow even faster collection of data.

With scan times as short as 30 seconds, contrast could be imaged during the first pass after injection. Imaging vascular contrast is a race against time, because it becomes diluted by crossing capillary beds and is rapidly cleared by the kidneys. Using fast, helical CT angiography, images of the hepatic vessels could be obtained while they were most opacified, providing good spatial and contrast resolution of the hepatic vasculature.

ADVANTAGES OF CT ANGIOGRAPHY

CT angiography is less invasive than radiographic angiography and provides better angiographic detail. For radiographic angiography, the abdomen must be opened to catheterize a jejunal vein. This method outlines the main portal vein and any shunting vessels cranial to the injection site, but does not opacify the entire portal system for evaluation. CT is more sensitive to changes in radiographic density and so is able to detect good contrast enhancement of vessels with a peripheral injection of contrast. With a peripheral injection, contrast is diluted when passing through the capillary bed of the small intestine before entering the portal vein. This mild opacification is not readily detectable with plain radiographs but is very evident with CT. Injecting peripherally fills all of the portal vasculature with contrast so that each tributary and branch is visible.

CT also provides volumetric imaging of the portal and hepatic vasculature. The surrounding tissues do not obscure the hepatic vasculature when the volume is rendered in axial images. When scrolling through a stack of CT images, the reader can build a mental 3D image of the structure of the portal and hepatic veins. Scrolling through images in both directions allows one to follow each vessel of interest while remaining in a standard plane relative to the body axis. This helps clinicians and surgeons visualize the anatomy of the vessels in question. The data can also be presented using volumetric image display which can help to define the anatomical relationships.

Although ultrasound can be a valuable tool in diagnosing portosystemic shunts, it has inherent physical limitations and is dependent on operator skill. The portal vasculature is deep in the abdomen, and patients usually have a small liver that is located under the costal arch. There may be limited scan windows because of gastrointestinal gas and overlying anatomy. Each ultrasound image, or series of images, is of small size and oriented toward the vessel in question. It is difficult for those not operating the transducer to gain a mental image of the course of the abdominal vessels without seeing the entire regional volume and having a plane of reference. CT imaging is not limited by these factors.

Software is available to construct 3D volume models of the vascular tree. These can be helpful; however, the overlying organs and musculoskeletal structures can make these images difficult to interpret. In addition, the dilution of contrast once it reaches the portal vein can result in poor discrimination between tissue and vasculature when building the 3D model. Good volumetric models depend on a tight contrast bolus, accurate scan timing, and lack of motion artifact.

Maximum intensity projections (MIPs) highlight the contrast-enhanced vessels and can improve tissue-vessel contrast resolution. Thick slabs can also be generated from adding multiple slices together, which can show tortuous shunt vessels in a single axial image. Finally, reformatting the images in multiple planes is helpful in demonstrating complex anatomy. Many of these features are available on Digital Imaging and Communications in Medicine imaging software applications.

TECHNICAL ASPECTS OF CT ANGIOGRAPHY

Production of a diagnostic quality CT angiogram depends on the timing, contrast bolus, catheter placement, and stillness of the patient. If one or more of these factors is not correctly applied, the diagnostic accuracy of the scan is significantly decreased. The goal of the scan is to image the hepatic and portal vasculature at the time of maximum contrast opacification, with minimal artifact.

A quality CT angiogram depends on stillness of the patient. Animals must be in respiratory pause during the scan, either by using a breath hold or inducing a period of apnea. Breathing causes the liver to be displaced in a cranial-caudal direction by the diaphragm, and vessel segments will not match between slices. Hyperventilation prior to initiating the scan can help to lower CO_2 and reduce the breathing reflex with both strategies.

The slice thickness chosen is a compromise between maximizing spatial resolution and minimizing the scan time. For most dogs, 3 to 5 mm collimation works well. Using an overlapping reconstruction can help in maximizing continuity between vessels. With multislice helical scanners, the collimation can be set much lower with the same or faster scan time.

The contrast injection must be performed in a cephalic vein or a jugular vein in very small dogs. A hind limb injection introduces undiluted contrast into the caudal vena cava and produces high-density artifacts as it passes through the liver. These bright and dark streaks obscure the vascular detail and hinder interpretation.

In order to acquire images of the portal and hepatic vasculature, the CT images must be timed to coincide with the first pass of contrast through the vessels. The timing of contrast arrival in the portal system varies between individuals and becomes more delayed with increased body weight. There are two strategies to obtain a start time for a portal scan: a dynamic CT, or bolus-tracking software. Using a dynamic CT, a small dose of contrast (1/4 the total dose) is injected into a cephalic vein, and the scan is started at the same time. The dynamic CT images the same slice over time, so that the portal vein can be seen filling with contrast. To determine the delay in seconds between contrast injection and starting scanning, the number of slices between start and full opacification are counted and multiplied by tube rotation time. If performing a dual-phase scan to include the hepatic arterial phase, the same can be applied to the hepatic artery or aorta, which have very similar opacification times. Bolus tracking software is available on some CT machines to monitor the time of arrival of a full contrast injection and to automatically start the scan. In this case, no separate dynamic CT is necessary.

SINGLE- AND DUAL-PHASE CT ANGIOGRAPHY OF THE LIVER

The hepatic arteries and the portal veins supply blood to the liver in two phases. The arterial phase arrives first and contributes approximately 25% of hepatic blood supply in normal dogs. The end of the arterial phase is overlaid by the portal phase, which rises and plateaus (**Fig. 1**) and provides most of the hepatic blood supply. The timing of the filling of hepatic arteries and portal veins requires different scan start and end times for each phase.

To image the portal phase only, the start of the scan must correspond with filling of the portal veins. This can range from 25 to 40 seconds after injection, depending on the size of the dog. A dynamic scan, as described here, is essential to determine the delay between injection and starting the scan. Portal phase scans should begin at the diaphragm and continue to the pelvic inlet. The entire abdomen should be included to allow for following tortuous extrahepatic and multiple acquired extrahepatic shunts.

Dual-phase scans include the arterial and portal phases and are excellent for delineating the hepatic arteries and arterioportal fistulae. The first phase is timed to coincide with arterial opacification, usually between 5 and 10 seconds after injection, and is scanned from the porta hepatis to the diaphragm. The portal phase is scanned in the reverse direction, beginning at the time of portal opacification, from the diaphragm to the pelvic inlet.[11]

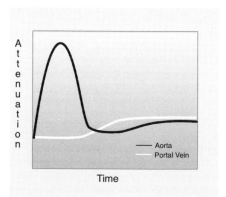

Fig. 1. Diagram of a time-attenuation curve of a contrast bolus and dynamic CT of the aorta and the portal vein. The liver is supplied with blood by the hepatic artery and the portal vein in two phases. The black curve represents the rapid contrast enhancement of the arterial system, which translates to hepatic artery opacification. After a rapid rise and fall, the portal vein attenuation rises gradually to a lesser degree and plateaus.

DIAGNOSING HEPATIC VASCULAR ANOMALIES

In order to use CT to diagnose hepatic vascular anomalies, one must be familiar with the normal anatomy of the portal and hepatic vasculature on cross-sectional imaging.[5,11] The appearance of the vessels on CT is very consistent between patients **(Fig. 2)**. The important arterial vessels include the celiac artery, hepatic artery, and gastroduodenal artery. Following the portal tributaries from caudal to cranial, the cranial and caudal mesenteric veins join to form the portal vein. The splenic vein enters from the left and the gastroduodenal vein from the right and ventral aspect, just cranial to the splenic vein. Cranial to this junction, the right branch of the portal vein supplies the right lateral and caudate lobes. The left branch travels cranially to give off a branch to the central liver division (right medial and quadrate lobes) and continues to the left liver lobes. The hepatic veins are branching structures in the cranial portion of the liver that interlace with the portal veins.

SINGLE EXTRAHEPATIC PORTOSYSTEMIC SHUNTS

Congenital single extrahepatic shunts are excellent candidates for CT. The abnormal vessel is usually large and easily delineated with contrast. The goals of interpreting the CT scan are to confirm the presence of a shunt, to describe its course, and to determine its origin and insertion **(Fig. 3A)**.

When initially searching for a shunt, tracing the portal tributaries is essential. Cranial to the point where the shunt originates from the portal vein or a tributary, the portal vein

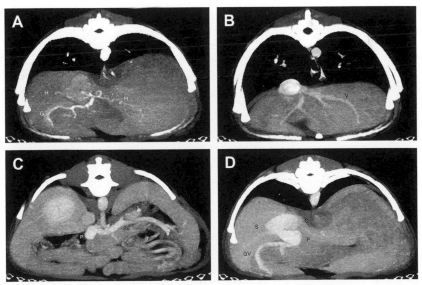

Fig. 2. Dual-phase CT angiography was used to generate thick-slab MIP images of a dog with a congenital right-divisional intrahepatic portosystemic shunt. The right of the animal is to the left of the image (*A–D*). (*A*) During the arterial phase, the enlarged hepatic arterial branches (H) and gastroduodenal artery (G) are visible. (*B*) The hepatic veins (V) are seen in the portal phase in the cranial portion of the liver. (*C*) The splenic vein (SV) is the large tributary joining the portal vein (P) on the left. (*D*) The gastroduodenal vein (GV) joins the portal vein ventrally from the right lobe of the pancreas. The large intrahepatic shunt (S) curves dorsally and cranially from the portal vein to the caudal vena cava (C).

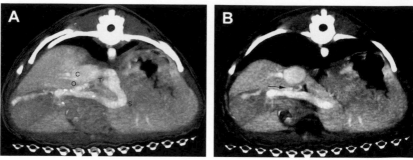

Fig. 3. Thick-slab MIP image of a dog with a congenital extrahepatic portosystemic shunt. (*A*) The thick slab MIP allows visualization of the entire shunt as it originates cranially and follows a tortuous route to the insertion caudally. The origin (O) is to the right of the portal vein, and the shunt (S) travels medially and then dorsally to the termination (T) in the caudal vena cava (C). (*B*) Cranial to the shunt origin, the portal vein (*arrow*) becomes small due to reduced blood flow. Only a portion of the shunt vessel is visible in this image.

diameter will decrease (**Fig. 3**B). This narrowing serves as a marker for the shunt origin. Common origins for single extrahepatic shunts are the portal vein just cranial to the splenic vein, the splenic vein, and the left gastric vein. The origin may not always be clearly seen if the vessel originates close to the splenic vein or if it is parallel to the scan plane. Partial volume artifact may average the two vessels together or render the vessel indistinct. CT conspicuity of the origin and insertion of extrahepatic shunts is otherwise excellent.[9]

The course of single extrahepatic shunts is variable. Left gastric vein shunts tend to travel dorsal to the fundus of the stomach and then run parallel to the diaphragm before inserting into the caudal vena cava cranial to the hepatic veins. These are particularly hard to diagnose with ultrasound, so they are very well suited to CT. Other shunts take a more direct route dorsally from the region of the porta hepatis or the splenic vein to the caudal vena cava. The variation in size and tortuosity of the abnormal vessels is considerable.

Single extrahepatic shunts most often insert into the caudal vena cava. This may be caudal or cranial to the liver. Once the origin of the shunt is located, it can be traced to the insertion point. A small proportion of shunts terminate in the azygos vein, which is located dorsal and to the right of the aorta. This results in a greatly enlarged azygos vein and may also be associated with other anomalies such as discontinuous caudal vena cava. The normal intrahepatic portal vein branches are small and may or may not be opacified with contrast.

INTRAHEPATIC PORTOSYSTEMIC SHUNTS

Large-breed dogs are more prone to congenital intrahepatic portosystemic shunts. In these cases, surgical planning depends on whether the shunt is left, central, or right divisional.[12] CT angiography provides optimal visualization of the vessel and allows for accurate classification (see **Fig. 2**). CT is also helpful in measuring the diameter of the shunt and caudal vena cava in cases where it will be repaired using an intravascular occlusion device and/or stent.

The portal tributaries generally appear normal in dogs with intrahepatic shunts. If a dual-phase scan is performed, there is often increased arterial contrast enhancement as the hepatic arteries make up the deficit of portal flow.[13] The hepatic arteries will be larger than normal and can cause a marbled appearance of the hepatic paren-chyma in the early phase. Within the liver, the intrahepatic shunt is of large diameter.

Right-divisional shunts deviate to the right lobes and can be somewhat tortuous as they meet the hepatic veins (see **Fig. 2**). A left-divisional shunt will travel left into the left medial lobe and then curve back toward the hepatic veins (**Fig. 4**). It often joins the left hepatic veins near the first branch. Central-divisional shunts travel in a relatively straight line through the liver parenchyma to the hepatic veins and tend to have a dilated ampulla terminally. The anatomically normal portal branches are small or absent.

MULTIPLE ACQUIRED EXTRAHEPATIC PORTOSYSTEMIC SHUNTS

Multiple acquired extrahepatic portosystemic shunts are formed secondary to portal hypertension from many causes including cirrhosis, thrombosis, and post-shunt liga-tion. Multiple small collateral vessels form, connecting the portal vein or its tributaries to the caudal vena cava. These are the most challenging CT scans to interpret, as the size and variability of the vessels are the greatest. These may also travel in any direc-tion in the abdomen, as far caudally as the bladder neck. It is critical to include the entire abdomen to diagnose these shunts.

One of the most common places for multiple acquired shunts to form is between the portal vein and the left renal vein. The vessels are often small in diameter and may appear as a blush or small strands of contrast enhancement. Larger vessels may orig-inate from the portal vein itself or from the splenic vein and join the caudal vena cava after a tortuous course. To follow these, one must scroll back and forth through the image stack as the vessel moves in and out of plane.

ARTERIOPORTAL FISTULAE

Arterioportal fistulae are rare congenital communications between the hepatic artery and the intrahepatic portal branches. The high-pressure flow causes dilation of the

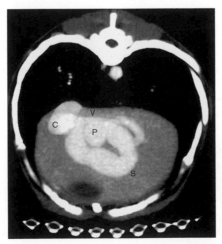

Fig. 4. Thick-slab MIP image of a dog with a congenital left-divisional intrahepatic portosys-temic shunt. The shunt originates from the left side of the portal vein (P) and then curves ventrally and cranially. It then travels dorsally to terminate in the left side of the caudal vena cava (C) near the entry of the hepatic veins (V).

portal veins, portal hypertension, and hepatofugal flow and formation of multiple extra-hepatic portosystemic shunts. These animals usually present at a young age with marked ascites, so they are clinically or ultrasonographically suspected to have a fistula. Dual-phase CT angiography can diagnose filling of the portal veins during the arterial phase for a definitive diagnosis and provide good vascular anatomical detail.

During a normal arterial phase, the liver parenchyma opacifies, and the hepatic arteries are visible parallel to the portal veins. In the case of a fistula, there is immediate filling of the portal veins with high-attenuating contrast from the arterial system (100–250 HU) (**Fig. 5**A). In normal dogs and those with portosystemic shunts, the portal veins enhance after 25 to 40 seconds and by approximately 40 HU, as the contrast is diluted in capillary beds. This immediate enhancement in the case of a fistula outlines the dilated and tortuous intrahepatic portal vein branches, which may protrude beyond the hepatic parenchyma. The liver itself is very small. In addition, usually multiple acquired extrahepatic portosystemic shunts form secondary to the hepatofugal flow and portal hypertension (**Fig. 5**B).

In rare cases, the communication is a low-flow system, and the entire portal system does not fill immediately.[8] These dogs tend to be older and suspected of having a congenital portosystemic shunt. Dual-phase CT angiography is necessary to determine the presence of a fistula in these dogs.

ADDITIONAL FINDINGS

Although the main goal of the scan is to delineate the portosystemic shunt, it is also important to be alert for other pathology, especially in dogs with multiple acquired shunts. Thrombosis of the portal or splenic veins can result in multiple extrahepatic shunts and can be diagnosed on CT. The thrombi appear as filling defects within the contrast-enhanced vessel.

Scans performed postsurgical correction of shunts can also demonstrate multiple acquired shunts and surgical implants. If it is questionable whether an attenuated extrahepatic vessel is still shunting, a dynamic CT can be performed distal to the ligation site to detect opacification. This determination can be difficult if the ligation is close to the caudal vena cava. The caudal vena cava fills with contrast earlier than

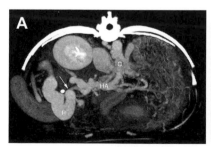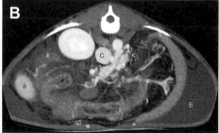

Fig. 5. Dual-phase CT angiography was used to generate thick-slab MIP images of a dog with a congenital arterioportal fistula. (*A*) During the arterial phase, the high-attenuating celiac artery (C) leads to the hepatic artery (HA), which is enlarged and tortuous. There is a connection between a hepatic artery branch and the intrahepatic portal vein branch (*arrow*). The portal vein branches are dilated and tortuous due to the high pressure and flow rate. (*B*) The portal hypertension results in peritoneal effusion (E) and multiple extrahepatic porto-systemic shunts (<) that lead to the caudal vena cava (C).

the portal vein because of venous contribution from the kidneys, and cannot be used to determine continued shunting.

Postsurgical ligation of intrahepatic shunts may also reveal enlarged, tortuous portal vessels within the parenchyma.[14] These need to be investigated further to determine whether they are shunting vessels or simply dilated portal vessels or hepatic veins.

Although the main goal of a CT scan in portal vascular anomalies is to depict the vascular anatomy, there is functional information available for interpretation as well. The dynamic CT scan used for determining scan timing can be evaluated with perfusion software to quantify the contribution of hepatic and arterial perfusion to total liver perfusion. Dogs with portosystemic shunts have a significantly greater proportion of arterial blood supply than portal blood supply, (hepatic perfusion index 0.59 +/−0.34) compared to normal dogs (hepatic perfusion index 0.19 +/−0.07).[13] The hepatic arteries are able to compensate for the reduced portal blood to maintain normal total perfusion. The volumetric nature of a CT scan also allows calculation of liver volume with appropriate software. Liver volume is reduced in dogs with portosystemic shunts, and increased after successful shunt ligation.[15] Both hepatic perfusion changes and hepatic volume measurements could serve as biomarkers for improved liver function post-surgery.

SUMMARY

CT angiography is a volumetric imaging method that is very well suited to diagnosing hepatic vascular anomalies. Abnormal vessels can be discovered and traced from their origin to their termination in the systemic circulation. Separate phases of the angiogram can be imaged to evaluate the arterial and portal phases of hepatic vascular flow. Detailed axial images and additional techniques such as 3D volume rendering and thick-slab MIPs can be used to demonstrate the abnormal vessel along its entire course. Single extrahepatic shunts, intrahepatic shunts, multiple acquired extrahepatic shunts, and arterioportal fistulae can all be diagnosed with this technique.

REFERENCES

1. Wrigley RH, Park RD, Konde LJ, et al. Subtraction portal venography. Vet Radiol 1987;28:208–12.
2. Koblik PD, Hornof WJ. Transcolonic sodium pertechnetate Tc 99m scintigraphy for diagnosis of macrovascular portosystemic shunts in dogs, cats, and potbellied pigs: 176 cases (1988–1992). J Am Vet Med Assoc 1995;207:729–33.
3. Lamb CR. Ultrasonographic diagnosis of congenital portosystemic shunts in dogs: results of a prospective study. Vet Radiol Ultrasound 1996;37:281–8.
4. Seguin B, Tobias KM, Gavin PR, et al. Use of magnetic resonance angiography for diagnosis of portosystemic shunts in dogs. Vet Radiol Ultrasound 1999;40: 251–8.
5. Frank P, Mahaffey M, Egger C, et al. Helical computed tomographic portography in ten normal dogs and ten dogs with a portosystemic shunt. Vet Radiol Ultrasound 2003;44:392–400.
6. Winter MD, Kinney LM, Kleine LJ. Three-dimensional helical computed tomographic angiography of the liver in five dogs. Vet Radiol Ultrasound 2005;46: 494–9.
7. Thompson MS, Graham JP, Mariani CL. Diagnosis of a porto-azygous shunt using helical computed tomography angiography. Vet Radiol Ultrasound 2003;44: 287–91.

8. Zwingenberger AL, McLear RC, Weisse C. Diagnosis of arterioportal fistulae in four dogs using computed tomographic angiography. Vet Radiol Ultrasound 2005;46:472–7.

9. Zwingenberger AL, Schwarz T, Saunders HM. Helical computed tomographic angiography of canine portosystemic shunts. Vet Radiol Ultrasound 2005;46: 27–32.

10. Bertolini G, Rolla EC, Zotti A, et al. Three-dimensional multislice helical computed tomography techniques for canine extra-hepatic portosystemic shunt assessment. Vet Radiol Ultrasound 2006;47:433–9.

11. Zwingenberger AL, Schwarz T. Dual-phase CT angiography of the normal canine portal and hepatic vasculature. Vet Radiol Ultrasound 2004;45:117–24.

12. Lamb CR. Ultrasonography of portosystemic shunts in dogs and cats. Vet Clin North Am Small Anim Pract 1998;28:725–53.

13. Zwingenberger AL, Shofer FS. Dynamic computed tomographic quantitation of hepatic perfusion in dogs with and without portal vascular anomalies. Am J Vet Res 2007;68:970–4.

14. Mehl ML, Kyles AE, Case JB, et al. Surgical management of left-divisional intra-hepatic portosystemic shunts: outcome after partial ligation of, or ameroid ring constrictor placement on, the left hepatic vein in twenty-eight dogs (1995–2005). Vet Surg 2007;36:21–30.

15. Stieger SM, Zwingenberger A, Pollard RE, et al. Hepatic volume estimation using quantitative computed tomography in dogs with portosystemic shunts. Vet Radiol Ultrasound 2007;48:409–13.

Scintigraphic Diagnosis of Portosystemic Shunts

Gregory B. Daniel, DVM, MS

KEYWORDS

- Portosystemic shunt • Radionuclide imaging • Diagnosis
- Portal scintigraphy • Technetium

Portosystemic shunts are vascular anomalies resulting in direct vascular communication between the portal venous system and the systemic venous circulation. The portal venous system drains the gastrointestinal track, pancreas, and spleen. The liver receives the portal blood and removes endogenous and exogenous toxins before they enter the systemic circulation. Portosystemic shunts allow portal blood to directly enter the systemic venous circulation, bypassing the liver. Animals with portosystemic shunts can have hepatic encephalopathy, chronic gastrointestinal signs, lower urinary tract signs, coagulopathies, and retarded growth.[1] These clinical signs are due to endogenous and exogenous toxins that are normally removed by the liver. Portosystemic shunts are classified as congenital or acquired.[2] Congenital portosystemic shunts are typically single macrovascular connections between the portal venous system and the caudal vena cava or other systemic veins, such as the azygos vein.[3,4] Congenital portosystemic shunts are further divided into intrahepatic and extrahepatic varieties.[5–7] Congenital intrahepatic portosystemic shunts occur mainly in large breed dogs and are described as left-, central-, or right-divisional branch shunts depending on their location within the liver.[6–8] There is a fairly equal incidence in the prevalence of the three types of intrahepatic shunts.[9] Left-divisional branch shunts are usually associated with a patent ductus venosus.[10] Irish wolfhounds have a higher incidence of left-divisional branch shunts.[11] Other breeds such as Old English Sheepdogs, Golden and Labrador Retrievers, and Australian Cattle Dogs have a higher incidence of central-divisional shunts.[12,13] Congenital extrahepatic portosystemic shunts are typically found in small breed dogs, such as Yorkshire Terrier, Miniature Schnauzer, Miniature Poodle, Shih Tzu, Lhasa Apso, Bichon Frise, and Cairn Terrier.[8] These shunts vary in location and typically terminate into the caudal vena cava or azygos vein.[3,4,14]

Department of Small Animal Clinical Sciences, Virginia-Maryland Regional College of Veterinary Medicine, Duckpond Drive, Phase II, Virginia Tech University, Blacksburg, VA 24061, USA
E-mail address: gdaniel@vt.edu

Vet Clin Small Anim 39 (2009) 793–810
doi:10.1016/j.cvsm.2009.04.009
0195-5616/09/$ – see front matter © 2009 Elsevier Inc. All rights reserved.

Acquired portosystemic shunts develop secondary to chronic portal hypertension.[15-17] Diseases such as idiopathic hepatic fibrosis have been shown to result in the development of acquired shunts.[15] Portal hypertension may also occur in young dogs secondary to congenital anomalies, such as portal vein atresia or hepatic arterioportal fistula.[5] Acquired portosystemic shunts take the form of multiple, small, torturous, extrahepatic shunt vessels that are found in the omentum or retroperitoneum near the left kidney, rectum, or esophagus.[7,14] These acquired extrahepatic portosystemic shunts will drain directly or indirectly into the caudal vena cava or other systemic veins.

The diagnosis of portosystemic shunts is first suspected based on history and physical findings with laboratory abnormalities.[18,19] The history may include signs of hepatoencephalopathy, with the owners recognizing incoordination, head pressing, disorientation, behavioral changes, seizures, depression and dementia.[20] Other findings can include stunted growth, polyuria and polydipsia, vomiting, blindness, and ptyalism in cats.[21-26] These findings are often exacerbated after feeding a high-protein meal. On physical examination, the animal may be small in stature and have a poor body condition. There is often a poor unkempt haircoat. The kidneys may palpate as enlarged. Non-Oriental breed cats may have a copper-colored iris.[27,28] The animal will have elevated paired preprandial and 2-hour postprandial bile acid levels.[29] Hyperammonemia is common, and ammonium biurate crystals may be found in the urine.[22,26,30] The animals will often have decreased blood urea nitrogen and hypoalbuminemia.[23]

The diagnosis of portosystemic shunt is confirmed by diagnostic imaging. Methods include survey radiographs, radiographic contrast procedures, ultrasound, (including Doppler color-flow and pulsed-wave Doppler sonography), computed tomography (CT), magnetic resonance imaging, or scintigraphy.[3,7,29,31-34] Survey radiographic findings include a small liver, renomegaly, occasionally ascites, or mineralized urate calculi. Ultrasonography (US) is now widely available in veterinary practices and is the most common method of imaging diagnosis of portosystemic shunts. Ultrasound can evaluate abdominal structures such as the liver and urinary system, which can be primarily or secondarily affected by the portosystemic shunt. Ultrasound can document the aberrant shunt vessel and has been used as a screening method for evaluation of dogs with congenital portosystemic shunts.[6,35-37] Changes in portal venous and caudal vena caval Doppler waveforms and color flow patterns have been described.[5,6,38,39] Nonmineralized cystic calculi, renomegaly, and a small liver with a reduced number and diameter of the portal vein at the level of the porta hepatis are common findings in ultrasound, suggestive of portosystemic shunts.[5,40] In dogs and cats with acquired portosystemic shunts secondary to portal hypertension, there is often ascites and the liver will have increased echogenicity with irregular margins. Color-flow Doppler imaging can be used to document multiple small shunting vessels in and around the renal vessels or the caudal abdominal retroperitoneum.[41] Ultrasound evaluation of the patient with a suspected portosystemic shunt can be time consuming, but in the hands of an experienced sonographer, it can have very high accuracy.[5,6]

Contrast mesenteric portovenograms provide reliable anatomic information, but the procedure is invasive and requires general anesthesia, selective catheter placement, contrast administration, and fluoroscopic imaging.[42,43] CT angiography also requires general anesthesia but only a peripheral intravenous injection of contrast medium. CT has the advantage of providing a three-dimensional representation of portal and hepatic vasculature.[44-46] Dual-phase intravenous CT angiography with a single-slice helical scanner has been used to image the hepatic and portal vasculature in normal dogs and dogs with portosystemic shunts.[32,47,48] Percutaneous injection of contrast medium into the splenic parenchyma as an alternative technique for CT portography has been described in humans and dogs.[49,50] A complete discussion of CT portography is found in the article by Zwingenberger elsewhere in this issue.

MRI has also been used to diagnosis portosystemic shunt. Magnetic resonance angiography has 80% sensitivity and 100% specificity for diagnosing portosystemic shunt. It can identify both single congenital shunts and multiple extrahepatic shunts.[34] The major drawback is the expense of the study and the general anesthesia requirement.

PORTAL SCINTIGRAPHY USING [99M] TC-SULFUR COLLOID

Scintigraphy has been used to evaluate dogs and cats for portosystemic shunting since the early 1980s. The first studies used ^{99m}Tc-sulfur colloid, which are small colloidal particles that localize within the reticuloendothelial system.[51,52] In the normal dog, the majority of the ^{99m}Tc-sulfur colloid will localize in the liver. In dogs with portosystemic shunts, a significant portion of the ^{99m}Tc-sulfur colloid will localize in the lung **(Fig. 1)**.[52–54] This technique is not specific to portosystemic shunts, because lung activity can also be seen in dogs with other causes of hepatic insufficiency, yet there is a strong association of decreased hepatic localization of ^{99m}Tc-sulfur colloid and portosystemic shunts.[52] ^{99m}Tc-sulfur colloid cannot be used in the cat for the diagnosis of portosystemic shunt, because lung uptake is seen in normal cats.[55]

The liver uptake of ^{99m}Tc-sulfur colloid principally reflects effective liver blood flow. Scintigraphy can be used to evaluate hepatic arterial and portal venous blood flow to the liver based on the first passage of the ^{99m}Tc-sulfur colloid in the liver.[52,53,56] These studies require a rapid series of images of the liver following a bolus injection of ^{99m}Tc-sulfur colloid **(Fig. 2)**. A time-activity plot of liver radioactivity is created from the series of images. The liver time-activity plot has two distinct phases or slopes. The relative volume of hepatic arterial and portal venous blood flow to the liver can be determined from the arterial and venous slopes of the hepatic time-activity plot. The first slope represents hepatic arterial flow, and the second slope represents the portal venous flow. The hepatic perfusion index is the ratio of the venous hepatic arterial slope over the portal slope. A normal dog will have similar slopes for the arterial and portal phases, and the hepatic arterial slope/portal slope (HPI) is 0.9 ± 0.4 (mean $\pm$ SD).[53] In an animal with a portosystemic shunt, there will be reduced portal flow relative to the arterial blood flow, and this will result in a elevated HPI of 6.7 ± 4.8 (mean $\pm$ SD).[53]

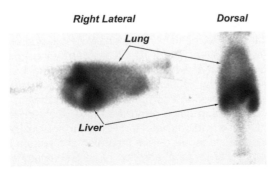

Fig. 1. Right lateral and dorsal views of a dog with a portosystemic shunt. Images were acquired 20 minutes following injection of ^{99m}Tc-sulfur colloid. The liver is smaller than normal, and there is diffuse uptake of the radiopharmaceutical within the lungs.

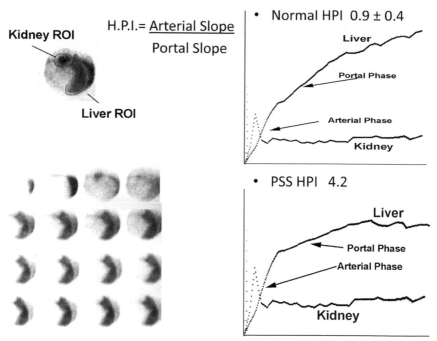

Fig. 2. Calculation of the hepatic perfusion index requires a dynamic image acquisition immediately following a bolus injection of a radiopharmaceutical such as ^{99m}Tc-sulfur colloid. The images at the lower left are right lateral images taken at a frame rate of 1 frame every 4 seconds. The image at the upper left is a composite image created by summing the images of the dynamic acquisition. Regions of interest are drawn around the kidney and liver. The graph in the upper right is of a normal dog, and the graph in the lower right is from a dog with a portosystemic shunt. There is decreased portal blood flow in the dog with the portosystemic shunt results in a shallower slope of the portal phase and thus an elevated hepatic perfusion index.

PER-RECTAL PORTAL SCINTIGRAPHY

Per-rectal portal scintigraphy (PRPS) was introduced in the 1990s.[33,57,58] This technique replaced other methods of nuclear imaging for diagnosis of portosystemic shunts as it was noninvasive, quick, inexpensive, easy to perform, and both highly sensitive and specific. Images of the portal venous system are made following administration of a radionuclide into the colon.[33,57–61] A lubricated red rubber feeding tube is placed into the distal colon to the level of the pelvic inlet (iliac crest) (**Fig. 3**). A three-way stopcock is used to connect a 6- or 10-mL air-filled syringe to the feeding tube. A shielded syringe containing the radionuclide (volume of 0.5 to 1.5 mL) is attached to the open port of the three-way stopcock. The computer acquisition is initiated, and the radionuclide is then pushed through the red rubber catheter. The radionuclide is deposited into the descending colon using the bolus of air. In veterinary medicine, the most commonly used radionuclide for PRPS is sodium pertechnetate (Na$^+$ ^{99m}TcO$_4^-$). Pertechnetate is absorbed from the colon and rectum and enters into the portal venous system.[62] Per-rectal absorption of pertechnetate in the normal dog is 15.26 ± 6.88% (mean ± SD) at 2 minutes.[63] In the normal animal, pertechnetate will flow with the blood traveling through the portal venous system into the liver (**Figs. 4** and **5**). There is no significant uptake or retention of pertechnetate by the liver, so

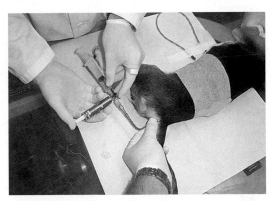

Fig. 3. PRPS is performed by administering the radionuclide into the distal colon. A lubricated red rubber feeding tube is advanced into the distal colon. A three-way stopcock is used to connect a 12-mL air-filled syringe and a shielded syringe containing the radionuclide. The position of a Co-57 marker can be seen ventral to the thorax/abdomen.

the majority of the pertechnetate will pass through the liver within 8 to 12 seconds. The pertechnetate is then noted within the heart.

In a dog or cat with portosystemic shunt, the portal blood containing the pertechnetate will bypass the liver and will be seen in the heart first (see **Figs 4** and **5**). The liver is

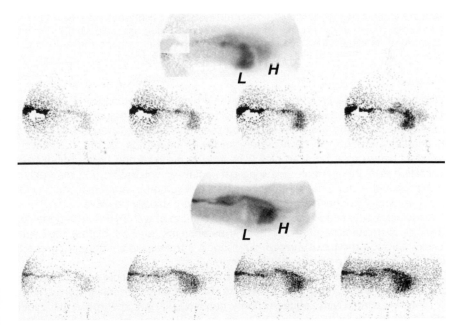

Fig. 4. PRPS in a normal dog (*top*) and a dog with a portoazygous shunt (*bottom*). The four images represent frames taken at 4 seconds each, and the single image is a composite created by summing 4 minutes of data. Note in the normal dog, the radionuclide is absorbed into the portal venous system and is delivered to the liver (*L*), then 8–12 seconds later, to the heart (*H*). In the dog with the portosystemic shunt, the radionuclide bypasses the liver (*L*) and delivers the radionuclide to the heart (*H*) first.

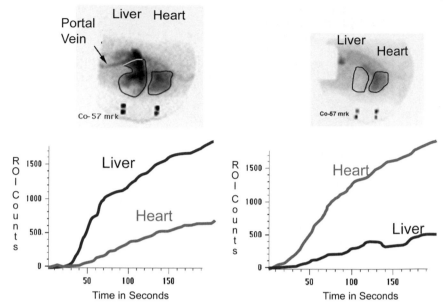

Fig. 5. PRPS in a normal dog (*left*) and a dog with a portocaval shunt (*right*). The images at the top are composite images created by summing the image of the dynamic acquisition. Note that the position of the Co-57 markers ventral to the dog helps identify the location of the heart and liver. Regions of interest are drawn around the liver and the heart. These regions are applied to the individual frames of the dynamic acquisition to create the time-activity curves shown at the bottom. Note that the normal dog has radioactivity within the liver before the heart, whereas, in the dog with the portosystemic shunt, the radioactivity is seen in the heart before the liver.

typically seen 10 to 12 seconds following the arrival of the radionuclide in the heart. Since most portosystemic shunts are of high magnitude, the majority of portal blood bypasses the liver, and the liver will not be seen until there is arterial delivery of the pertechnetate through the celiac artery. In lower-magnitude shunts, the arrival of the pertechnetate may be seen simultaneously in the liver and heart. Shunt vessel visualization is highly variable following per-rectal administration and may only be possible when the study has been reformatted and summed. Anatomic characterization of the type of congenital or acquired shunt is not usually possible.

Dogs with microvascular dysplasia will appear normal with PRPS. The pertechnetate will be distributed throughout the liver parenchyma and will bypass the hepatic sinusoids through the thousands of microscopic intrahepatic shunts, giving one the impression of normal perfusion of the liver.

Dogs with acquired portosystemic shunts typically have multiple small vessels, but these are rarely seen on per-rectal portal studies. Portal hypertension, which is typically found in animals with acquired shunts, can result in poor absorption of the radionuclide from the colon.

Correct identification of the liver and the heart can be difficult in small patients or in patients with poor colonic absorption of the pertechnetate. External radioactive markers can be used to identify the position of the liver and heart. One marker is positioned ventral to the xiphoid process of the caudal sternum for marking hepatic position, and the other marker is placed ventral to the apex beat of the heart (see

Figs. 3 and 5). External markers are especially helpful in cases of poor radionuclide absorption by the colon/rectum.

Quantitative analysis of the PRPS is possible using an imaging computer. The computer estimates the percentage of portal blood that bypasses the liver.[55,58] The shunt fraction (SF) is calculated from the integral counts in the heart and liver during the 12-second period of normal liver transit using the following formula:

$$\text{Shunt Fraction} = \frac{\sum_n \text{Heart Counts}}{\sum_n \text{Heart Counts} + \sum_n \text{Liver Counts}}$$

where n = 12 seconds.

The total number of counts for the heart is divided by the sum of the total counts for the heart and liver and is reported as a percentage. Normal dogs should have a SF of less than 5%. If there is poor or slow absorption of the radionuclide, the SF may be as high as 15% to 20% in normal dogs and cats. Most cases of congenital portosystemic shunts will have SFs greater than 60%. The typical SF value for congenital portosystemic shunts will be between 80% and 95%.

Quantification of the SF has been shown by some investigators to be a reliable method for assessment of shunt attenuation following surgery.[58,60,64] Others have shown that measurements of SF values are not reproducible between operators.[65] In either case, SF values have no prognostic significance and will not predict how an animal will respond to surgical intervention for intrahepatic shunts.[66] In a review of 110 portosystemic shunt cases performed at the University of Tennessee, no correlations were found between the SF values and serum ammonia levels, age of the animal, serum blood urea nitrogen levels, total protein, albumin, preligation intraportal pressure, or postligation intraportal pressure at the time of surgery.[55]

Some dogs will have a nonuniform distribution of the radionuclide within the liver following per-rectal administration. Blood flows though the portal venous system in discrete channels. This laminar flow pattern prevents homogeneous mixing of the radionuclide within the portal vein, resulting in a streamline flow pattern and nonuniform distribution in the liver. There are three patterns of nonuniform distribution of the radionuclide recognized: dorsal hepatic distribution, central hepatic distribution (porta hepatis), and ventral hepatic distribution (**Fig. 6**).[67] This occurs as the radionuclide selectively flows into one of the three branches of the portal vein. The right-divisional branch of the portal vein supplies portal venous blood to the caudate, right lateral, and right medial hepatic lobes, and streamlining into this branch results in a dorsal hepatic distribution as seen on a lateral view. If the radioactivity is confined primarily to the central-divisional branch, then the radioactivity will distribute to the central hepatic lobes, and the radioactivity will have a central hepatic distribution on a lateral view. If the radioactivity is confined primarily to the left-divisional branch, then the radioactivity will be distributed to the left hepatic lobes and will have a ventral distribution on the lateral view. The nonuniform distribution of the radionuclide within the liver should not be interpreted as abnormal but as a variation of normal portal blood flow.

The main disadvantage of PRPS is that morphologic descriptions of the shunt are usually not possible, and, sometimes, the studies are nondiagnostic. The accuracy of interpretation is dependent on the quality of the study. The primary reason for a poor or nondiagnostic study is poor absorption of the radionuclide from the colon. A relatively large amount (10–20 mCi, 370–740 MBq) of $^{99m}\text{TcO}_4$ is administered to help overcome the limitations of poor absorption. If the administration site within the colon is in the image field of view, the image quality is degraded due to excessive

Right	Central	Left

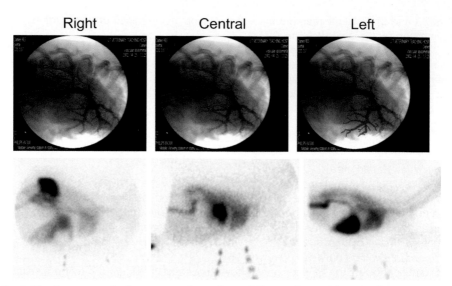

Fig. 6. The images at the bottom are from three different dogs with normal portal venous systems. There is focal distribution of the radionuclide in the dorsal, central, and ventral aspects of the liver due to streamlining of the radionuclide into the right-, central-, and left-divisional branches of the portal vein. The images at the top are portal venograms showing the selective distribution in the right-, central-, and left-divisional branches of the portal vein.

background activity created by the "bloom" at the deposition site, making it difficult to see the lower-intensity areas of the heart and liver.

TRANS-SPLENIC INJECTION OF $^{99M}TCO_4$

Ultrasound-guided trans-splenic portal scintigraphy was developed to overcome many of the disadvantages of PRPS.[3,4,63] Trans-splenic portal scintigraphy is easy and rapid to perform and provides a nuclear scintigram of the portal vasculature. The radiopharmaceutical is absorbed quickly from the splenic parenchyma, with a much higher percentage of the injected does entering the portal venous system (52.5 ± 19.06% for trans-splenic portal scintigraphy versus 9.23 ± 5.66% for PRPS [mean±DS]).[63] The resulting images are higher in quality compared with PRPS.[3,63]

A 7.5-MHz or 8.0-MHz micro convex ultrasound probe is used to locate the spleen and guide the injection of the radiopharmaceutical (**Fig. 7**). A 1.5-in, 22-gauge needle is used to administer the radiopharmaceutical into the spleen. It is not necessary to inject the radiopharmaceutical directly into a splenic vein but instead into a central region of the splenic parenchyma. Absorption of the radiopharmaceutical from the spleen is fast, so the computer must be set to acquire a frame rate of four frames per second. The images are evaluated both visually and quantitatively.

In the normal dog, the radiopharmaceutical is rapidly absorbed from the spleen into the splenic vein into the left gastric vein, and then into the main portal vein (**Fig. 8**). The total amount of absorption from the spleen is dependent on the injection technique, but typically more than 50% of the injected dose will enter the portal venous system. The radiopharmaceutical will outline the portal system, delivering the radioactivity to the liver first. The radiopharmaceutical will pass through the hepatic sinusoids to the

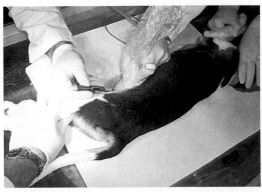

Fig. 7. Trans-splenic portal scintigraphy is performed by administering the radionuclide into the spleen via ultrasound guidance. The animal is placed in right lateral recumbency. The ultrasound transducer is held in the left hand, and the radionuclide, within a shielded syringe, is held with the right hand as the needle is advanced into the spleen.

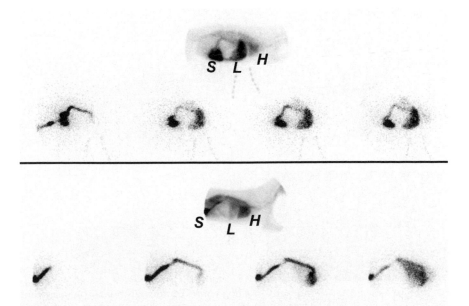

Fig. 8. Trans-splenic portal scintigraphy in a normal dog (*top*) and a dog with a portoazygous shunt (*bottom*). The four images represent frames taken at 2 seconds each, and the single image is a composite created by summing 4 minutes of data. The radionuclide was administered into the spleen (*S*). Note in the normal dog the radionuclide is absorbed into the portal venous system and is delivered to the liver (*L*), then 6–8 seconds later, to the heart (*H*). In the dog with the PSS, the radionuclide bypasses the liver (*L*) and delivers the radionuclide to the heart (*H*) first.

hepatic vein, caudal vena cava, and then to the heart. In the normal dog, the transit time from the liver to the heart is 7.03 ± 2.3 (mean ± SD) seconds.[63]

Image analysis is performed by creating a composite image of the image series. Regions of interest (ROIs) are drawn around the area of the heart and liver. The timing of the radiopharmaceutical arrival in the liver and heart is evaluated by superimposing the ROIs over a cinematic display of the image series.

Liver and heart time-activity curves are derived from the dynamic acquisition and used to calculate the SF. SFs are determined as with the per-rectal studies, but because radioactivity arrives in a more discrete bolus, hepatic transit time is shorter than that with PRPS. SF is determined using the following formula:

$$\text{Shunt Fraction} = \frac{\sum_n \text{Heart Counts}}{\sum_n \text{Heart Counts} + \sum_n \text{Liver Counts}}$$

where n = 7 seconds (the hepatic transit time in normal dogs). The SF for normal dogs is 2.64 ± 1.3.37.

The main advantage of trans-splenic portal scintigraphy over PRPS is the quality of the nuclear portovenogram, which permits visualization of a shunting vessel or vessels in more than 90% of the cases (**Figs. 9** and **10**).[3,63] However, there is a learning curve to performing these studies, and experience is associated with a decreased number of nondiagnostic studies. Most nondiagnostic studies (10.7%) result from intraperitoneal, rather than intrasplenic, administration of the radiopharmaceutical. When the spleen is very small, it is more challenging to place the needle in the splenic parenchyma and keep it in place during the injection. There is a higher probability of

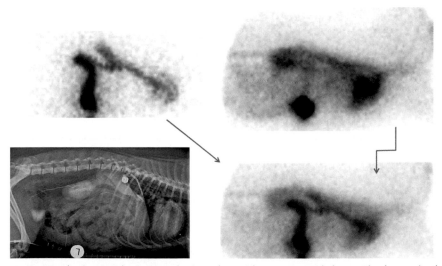

Fig. 9. Trans-splenic portal scintigraphy in a dog with a portocaval shunt. The image in the upper left is a composite image of the first passage of the radionuclide through the portovenous system. The image on the upper right is a composite image created by summing the entire dynamic series. The image on the lower right is a fusion image of the top two images showing the location of the shunt relative to the heart and liver. The image in the lower left is a contrast portovenogram following placement of an ameroid constrictor around a shunt vessel. The shunt persists following placement of the ameroid constrictor. Note that the portal scan shows the shunt deviated dorsally, then extending ventrally along the diaphragm, as shown on the contrast venogram.

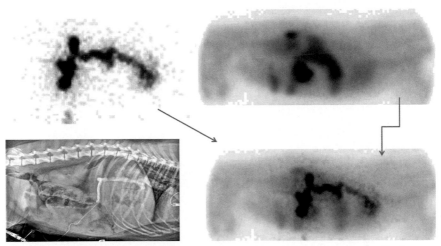

Fig. 10. Trans-splenic portal scintigraphy in a dog with an intrahepatic shunt. The image on the upper left is a composite image of the first passage of the radionuclide through the portovenous system. The image on the upper right is a composite image created by summing the entire dynamic series. The image on the lower right is a fusion image of the top two images showing the location of the shunt relative to the heart and liver. The image on the lower left is a contrast portovenogram. Note the ventral deviation of the shunt vessel within the liver parenchyma, which is seen on both the scintigraphic and contrast studies.

extravasation of the radiopharmaceutical outside the spleen when the needle is placed in a steep angle into the spleen or if it is inadvertently advanced completely through the spleen and subsequently withdrawn so that the tip of the needle was within the parenchyma before injection. Directing the needle in a shallow angle relative to the spleen will allow the tip of the needle to be further away from the point where the needle penetrated the splenic capsule. This inhibits the leakage of the radiopharmaceutical along the needle track. In cases where the needle is advanced too deeply in the spleen on the first attempt, better quality studies are achieved by finding a new location in the spleen. Injection speed may also play a role in the study quality: during a rapid injection through a small needle, it is possible that some of the radiopharmaceutical is forced along the needle tract and into the peritoneal cavity.

A potential limitation of the trans-splenic technique is the identification of portosystemic shunts located caudal to the entrance of the splenic vein into the portal vein. Most extrahepatic portosystemic shunts arise from the main portal vein, splenic vein, or the left gastric vein and empty into the caudal vena cava cranial to the phrenicoabdominal vein. These would not be missed with trans-splenic portal scintigraphy.[2,68] The portal hemodynamics cranial to the shunt have been documented as hepatofugal portal flow (flow in a caudal direction) by intraoperative ultrasound in a series of dogs.[38] Because the radioactive bolus will travel the path of least resistance and only a small quantity of radioactivity is needed to create the nuclear venoportogram, we have yet to see a false-negative study when the shunt is caudal to the left gastric vein. Another limitation of trans-splenic portal scintigraphy is that, as for per-rectal portal scintigraphy, negative results are likely to result in the presence of microvascular dysplasia.

In most cases of portosystemic shunts, the radiopharmaceutical bypasses the liver on the first pass, entering the systemic venous circulation, which delivers the radionuclide to the heart. The liver may not be seen until the radiopharmaceutical has entered

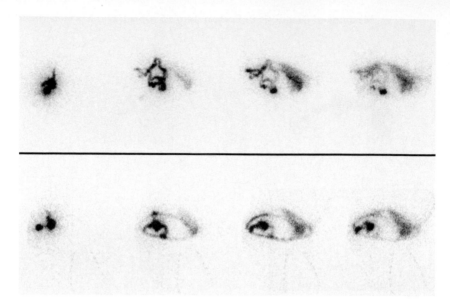

Fig. 11. Trans-splenic portal scintigraphy in two dogs with acquired portosystemic shunts. The dog in the top series has multiple shunt vessels that enter the caudal vena cava near the left kidney. The dog in the bottom series has multiple shunt vessels that enter the caudal vena cava near the rectum and left kidney. In addition, there are shunt vessels that terminate into the internal thoracic vein.

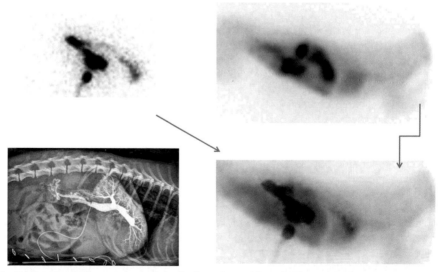

Fig. 12. Trans-splenic portal scintigraphy in a dog with multiple acquired shunts. The image on the upper left is a composite image of the first passage of the radionuclide through the portovenous system. The image on the upper right is a composite image created by summing the entire dynamic series. The image on the lower right is a fusion image of the top two images showing the location of the shunt relative to the heart and liver. The image on the lower left is a contrast portovenogram. In this case, the shunt vessels are too small to be resolved scintigraphically, but the hepatofugal flow of the radionuclide toward the kidney is indicative of acquired shunts.

through the hepatic arteries. The abnormal temporal sequence of organ visualization, heart before liver, is indicative of a portosystemic shunt. If the portosystemic shunt is of low magnitude, the liver may be seen simultaneously or slightly before the heart. Diagnosis of a portosystemic shunt is supported by a short hepatic transit time, that is, the length of time from the first arrival of the radiopharmaceutical in the liver until the radiopharmaceutical is seen in the heart. Calculated hepatic transit time in normal dogs was reported to range from 5.00 to 10.75 seconds with a mean of 7.03 seconds.[63] A hepatic transit time of less than 2 seconds is indicative of a portosystemic shunt.

Trans-splenic portal scintigraphy can determine the termination point of the portosystemic shunt into the systemic venous circulation. Three distinct shunt terminations have been identified; portoazygos, portocaval/splenocaval, and internal thoracic vessels.

Imaging characteristic seen on trans-splenic portoscintigraphy indicative of acquired shunts include visualization of more than one shunt vessel (**Fig. 11**). Multiple vessels are not always seen; however, one of the most common patterns observed with acquired shunts is hepatofugal flow of the radiopharmaceutical (**Fig. 12**).[69] In portoazygous shunts, the flow of the radiopharmaceutical is generally dorsal and then cranial following trans-splenic administration.[69] With some congenital shunts, there may be a slight caudal direction as the radiopharmaceutical passes through a long tortuous vessel, but the caudal extent does not go back as far as the kidneys.

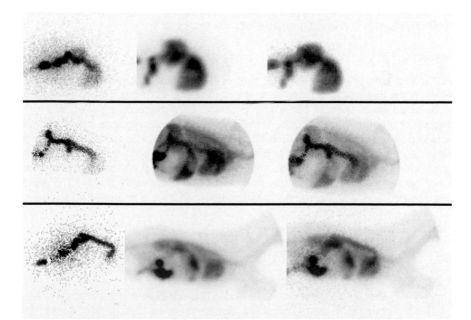

Fig. 13. Trans-splenic portal scintigraphy using ^{99m}Tc-mebrofenin in a normal dog (*top*), a dog with a portocaval shunt (*middle*), and a dog with a portoazygous shunt (*bottom*). The images on the left are images made during the first passage of the radiopharmaceutical. The central images are summed images of the entire dynamic acquisition. The images on the right are fused images of the first pass and the summed images. The ^{99m}Tc-mebrofenin localizes within the liver, making it easy to identify the location of the shunt vessel relative to the liver.

In small animals, most acquired portosystemic shunts result from opening of splenorenal and mesenteric collateral vessels. Less common location of acquired shunts can be through gastrophrenic, pancreaticoduodenal, and rarely hemorrhoidal collaterals. Because of portal hypertension, there will be enough hepatofugal flow for the scintigraphic diagnosis of a clinically significant portosystemic shunt even if it originates caudal to the splenic vein. Another suggestive finding is slow absorption and slow transit of the radiopharmaceutical through the portal venous system.

TRANS-SPLENIC INJECTION OF ^{99M}TC-MEBROFENIN

^{99m}Tc-mebrofenin can be used as an alternative to sodium pertechnetate for trans-splenic portal scintigraphy. The absorption of ^{99m}Tc-mebrofenin from the spleen is similar to pertechnetate, and both create excellent images of the portal vein. However, ^{99m}Tc-mebrofenin has a high first-pass extraction by the liver, which means that in a normal animal, only a small portion of the ^{99m}Tc-mebrofenin passes through the liver into the caudal vena cava and heart. The ^{99m}Tc-mebrofenin retained by the liver is gradually cleared into the biliary system with a clearance half-time of 19 minutes. In normal dogs, following trans-splenic injection of ^{99m}Tc-mebrofenin, radioactivity is confined to the liver. Dogs with portosystemic shunts have a conspicuously different pattern as ^{99m}Tc-mebrofenin bypasses the liver and is first seen in the heart (see **Fig. 1**). ^{99m}Tc-mebrofenin will eventually be extracted by the liver following hepatic arterial delivery. This is particularly useful in identifying the location of the shunt relative to the liver. By summing the images during with first passage of the radiopharmaceutical with a 5-minute static image of the liver, the location of the shunt is more easily identified (**Fig. 13**). This is not possible with pertechnetate.

SUMMARY

Portal scintigraphy provides a reliable, safe, and dependable diagnostic procedure for evaluating macroscopic portosystemic shunts in dogs and cats. Portal scintigraphy can be used as a primary screening procedure for portosystemic shunts or as a backup procedure to ultrasound. Trans-splenic portal scintigraphy can distinguish between portoazygos and portocaval/splenocaval shunts and, sometimes, between congenital versus acquired shunts. It does not, however, allow distinction between single intrahepatic and extrahepatic shunts. Trans-splenic portal scintigraphy in now the nuclear technique of choice for detection of portosystemic shunts. The advantages over PRPS include decreases in radiation exposure and improved image quality.

REFERENCES

1. Berent A, Weisse C. Portosystemic shunts and portal venous hypoplasia. Compendium on Standards of Care Emergency and Critical Care Medicine 2007;9(3):1–11.
2. Payne JT, Martin RA, Constantinescu GM. The anatomy and embryology of portosystemic shunts in dogs and cats. Semin Vet Med Surg (Small Anim) 1990; 5(2):75–82.
3. Morandi F, Cole RC, Tobias KM, et al. Use of 99mTCO4- trans-splenic portal scintigraphy for diagnosis of portosystemic shunts in 28 dogs. Vet Radiol Ultrasound 2005;46(2):153–61.
4. Sura PA, Tobias KM, Morandi F, et al. Comparison of 99mTcO4- trans-splenic portal scintigraphy with per-rectal portal scintigraphy for diagnosis of portosystemic shunts in dogs. Vet Surg 2007;36(7):654–60.

5. Lamb CR. Ultrasonography of portosystemic shunts in dogs and cats. Vet Clin North Am Small Anim Pract 1998;28(4):725–53.
6. Lamb CR. Ultrasonographic diagnosis of congenital portosystemic shunts in dogs: results of a prospective study. Vet Radiol Ultrasound 1996;37(4):281–8.
7. Lamb CR, Daniel GB. Diagnostic imaging of portosystemic shunts. Compend Contin Educ Vet 2002;24:626–35.
8. Hunt GB. Effect of breed on anatomy of portosystemic shunts resulting from congenital diseases in dogs and cats: a review of 242 cases. Aust Vet J 2004; 82(12):746–9.
9. Krotscheck U, Adin CA, Hunt GB, et al. Epidemiologic factors associated with the anatomic location of intrahepatic portosystemic shunts in dogs. Vet Surg 2007; 36(1):31–6.
10. Bahr A, Grevel V. Congenital portosystemic shunt in 56 dogs: signs, diagnostic evaluation and operation. Kleintierpraxis 2005;50(4):235–47.
11. Meyer HP, Rothuizen J, Ubbink GJ, et al. Increasing incidence of hereditary intra-hepatic portosystemic shunts in Irish Wolfhounds in the Netherlands (1984 to 1992). Vet Rec 1995;136(1):13–6.
12. Tisdall PLC, Hunt GB, Bellenger CR, et al. Congenital portosystemic shunts in Maltese and Australian cattle dogs. Aust Vet J 1994;71(6):174–8.
13. Hunt GB, Tisdall PLC, Webb A, et al. Congenital portosystemic shunts in toy and miniature poodles. Aust Vet J 2000;78(8):530–2.
14. Boothe HW, Howe LM, Edwards JF, et al. Multiple extrahepatic portosystemic shunts in dogs: 30 cases (1981–1993). J Am Vet Med Assoc 1996;208(11): 1849–54.
15. Rutgers HC, Haywood S, Kelly DF. Idiopathic hepatic fibrosis in 15 dogs. Vet Rec 1993;133(5):115–8.
16. Kim J, Han S, Chun H, et al. Diagnosis of multiple extrahepatic portosystemic shunt in two dogs. Journal of Veterinary Clinics 2007;24(2):269–75.
17. Langdon P, Cohn LA, Kreeger JM, et al. Acquired portosystemic shunting in two cats. J Am Anim Hosp Assoc 2002;38(1):21–7.
18. Tobias K. Diagnosis and management of portosystemic shunts - Part I. Presented at the Proceedings of the North American Veterinary Conference, Small animal and exotics. Orlando, FL, 2007.
19. Tobias K. Diagnosis and management of portosystemic shunts - Part II. Presented at the Proceedings of the North American Veterinary Conference, Small animal and exotics. Orlando, FL, 2007.
20. Wolschrijn CF, Mahapokai W, Rothuizen J, et al. Gauged attenuation of congenital portosystemic shunts: results in 160 dogs and 15 cats. Vet Q 2000;22(2):94–8.
21. Cape L, Panciera DL, Partington B, et al. Glomerulonephritis and a congenital por-tocaval shunt in a seven-year-old dog. J Am Anim Hosp Assoc 1992;28(5):419–24.
22. Bartges JW, Cornelius LM, Osborne CA. Ammonium urate uroliths in dogs with portosystemic shunts. In: Bonaqura JB, editor. Kirk's current veterinary therapy XIII: small animal practice. Philadelphia: WB Saunders; 2000. p. 872–4.
23. Cornelius CE. Biochemical evaluation of hepatic function in dogs. J Am Anim Hosp Assoc 1979;15(3):259–69.
24. Ewing GO, Suter PF, Bailey CS. Hepatic insufficiency associated with congenital anomalies of the portal vein in dogs. J Am Anim Hosp Assoc 1974;10(5):463–76.
25. Grauer GF, Pitts RP. Primary polydipsia in three dogs with portosystemic shunts. J Am Anim Hosp Assoc 1987;23(2):197–200.
26. Griffiths GL, Lumsden JH, Valli VEO. Hematologic and biochemical changes in dogs with portosystemic shunts. J Am Anim Hosp Assoc 1981;17(5):705–10.

27. Birchard SJ, Sherding RG. Portosystemic shunts. Feline Pract 1995;23(2):5–9.
28. Birchard SJ, Sherding RG. Feline portosystemic shunts. Compend Contin Educ Vet 1992;14(10):1295–300.
29. Burton CA, White RN. Portovenogram findings in cases of elevated bile acid concentrations following correction of portosystemic shunts. J Small Anim Pract 2001;42(11):536–40.
30. Meyer DJ, Strombeck DR, Stone EΛ, et al. Ammonia tolerance test in clinically normal dogs and in dogs with portosystemic shunts. J Am Vet Med Assoc 1978;173(4):377–9.
31. Meyer-Lindenberg A, Ebermaier C, Wolvekamp P, et al. Comparative evaluation of analog and digital radiographs of six different body-regions of the dog. Berliner und Münchener Tierärztliche Wochenschrift 2008;121(5/6):216–27.
32. Frank P, Mahaffey M, Egger C, et al. Helical computed tomographic portography in ten normal dogs and ten dogs with a portosystemic shunt. Vet Radiol Ultrasound 2003;44(4):392–400.
33. Daniel GB, Bright R, Ollis P, et al. Per rectal portal scintigraphy using [99m]technetium pertechnetate to diagnose portosystemic shunts in dogs and cats. J Vet Intern Med 1991;5(1):23–7.
34. Seguin B, Tobias KM, Gavin PR, et al. Use of magnetic resonance angiography for diagnosis of portosystemic shunts in dogs. Vet Radiol Ultrasound 1999; 40(3):251–8.
35. Holt DE, Schelling CG, Saunders HM, et al. Correlation of ultrasonographic findings with surgical, portographic, and necropsy findings in dogs and cats with portosystemic shunts: 63 cases (1987–1993). J Am Vet Med Assoc 1995; 207(9):1190–3.
36. Holt DE, Saunders HM, Schelling C, et al. Diagnosis of portosystemic shunts: correlation of ultrasound with surgical, portographic and necropsy findings 63 cases (1987–1993). Veterinary Surgery 1994;23:403.
37. d'Anjou MA. The sonographic search for portosystemic shunts. Clin Tech Small Anim Pract 2007;22(3):104–14.
38. Szatmári V, Sluijs FJv, Rothuizen J, et al. Ultrasonographic assessment of haemodynamic changes in the portal vein during surgical attenuation of congenital extrahepatic portosystemic shunts in dogs. J Am Vet Med Assoc 2004;224(3): 395–402.
39. Szatmári V, Sluijs FJv, Rothuizen J, et al. Intraoperative ultrasonography of the portal vein during attenuation of intrahepatic portocaval shunts in dogs. J Am Vet Med Assoc 2003;222(8):1086–92.
40. Santilli RA, Gerboni G, Olivieri M, et al. Ultrasonographic diagnosis of portosystemic shunts in dogs and cats: a retrospective study of 51 cases. Veterinaria (Cremona) 2003;17(2):13–23.
41. Salwei RM, O'Brien RT, Matheson JS. Use of contrast harmonic ultrasound for the diagnosis of congenital portosystemic shunts in three dogs. Vet Radiol Ultrasound 2003;44(3):301–5.
42. Wrigley RH, Park RD, Konde LJ, et al. Subtraction portal venography. Vet Radiol Ultrasound 1987;28(6):208–12.
43. Birchard SJ, Biller DS, Johnson SE. Differentiation of intrahepatic versus extrahepatic portosystemic shunts in dogs using positive-contrast portography. J Am Anim Hosp Assoc 1989;25(1):13–7.
44. Jung J, Chae W, Chang J, et al. Diagnostic imaging of portosystemic shunt using CT in two dogs. Journal of Veterinary Clinics 2007;24(3):461–6.

45. Zwingenberger AL, Shofer FS. Dynamic computed tomographic quantitation of hepatic perfusion in dogs with and without portal vascular anomalies. Am J Vet Res 2007;68(9):970–4.

46. Bertolini G, Rolla EC, Zotti A, et al. Three-dimensional multislice helical computed tomography techniques for canine extra-hepatic portosystemic shunt assessment. Vet Radiol Ultrasound 2006;47(5):439–43.

47. Zwingenberger AL, Schwarz T, Saunders HM. Helical computed tomographic angiography of canine portosystemic shunts. Vet Radiol Ultrasound 2005;46(1):27–32.

48. Thompson MS, Graham JP, Mariani CL. Diagnosis of a porto-azygous shunt using helical computed tomography angiography. Vet Radiol Ultrasound 2003;44(3):287–91.

49. Sawada S, Nakamura K, Tanigawa N, et al. Computed tomographic percutaneous transplenic portography. Acta Radiol 1993;34:529–31.

50. Echandi RL, Morandi F, Daniel WT, et al. Comparison of transplenic multidetector CT portography to multidetector CT-angiography in normal dogs. Vet Radiol Ultrasound 2007;48(1):38–44.

51. Daniel GB, Tucker RL. Liver scintigraphy - application in small animals. Semin Vet Med Surg (Small Anim) 1991;6(2):154–63.

52. Koblik PD, Hornof WJ. Technetium 99m sulfur colloid scintigraphy to evaluate reticuloendothelial system function in dogs with portasystemic shunts. J Vet Intern Med 1995;9(6):374–80.

53. Koblik PD, Hornof WJ, Breznock EM. Use of quantitative hepatic scintigraphy to evaluate spontaneous portosystemic shunts in 12 dogs. Vet Radiol Ultrasound 1983;24(5):232–5.

54. Hornof WJ, Koblik PD, Breznock EM. Radiocolloid scintigraphy as an aid to the diagnosis of congenital portacaval anomalies in the dog. J Am Vet Med Assoc 1983;182(1):44–6.

55. Daniel GB, Berry CR. Scintigraphic diagnosis of portosystemic shunts. In: Daniel GB, Berry CR, editors. Textbook of veterinary nuclear medicine. Harrisburg (PA): American College of Veterinary Radiology; 2006. p. 231–55.

56. Koblik PD, Hornof WJ, Breznock EM. Quantitative hepatic scintigraphy in the dog. Vet Radiol Ultrasound 1983;24(5):226–31.

57. Koblik PD, Komtebedde J, Yen CK, et al. Use of transcolonic 99mtechnetium-pertechnetate as a screening test for portosystemic shunts in dogs. J Am Vet Med Assoc 1990;196(6):925–30.

58. Daniel GB, Bright R, Monnet E, et al. Comparison of per-rectal portal scintigraphy using tc-99m pertechnetate to mesenteric injection of radioactive microspheres for quantification of portosystemic shunts in an experimental dog-model. Vet Radiol Ultrasound 1990;31(4):175–81.

59. Koblik PD, Yen CK, Hornof WJ, et al. Use of transcolonic 123I-Iodoamphetamine to diagnose spontaneous portosystemic shunts in 18 dogs. Vet Radiol Ultrasound 1989;30(2):67–73.

60. Vechten BJv, Komtebedde J, Koblik PD. Use of transcolonic portal scintigraphy to monitor blood flow and progressive postoperative attenuation of partially ligated single extrahepatic portosystemic shunts in dogs. J Am Vet Med Assoc 1994;204(11):1770–4.

61. Koblik PD, Hornof WJ. Transcolonic sodium pertechnetate Tc 99m scintigraphy for diagnosis of macrovascular portosystemic shunts in dogs, cats, and potbellied pigs: 176 cases (1988–1992). J Am Vet Med Assoc 1995;207(6):729–33.

62. Shiomi S, Kuroki T, Kurai O, et al. Portal circulation by technetium-99m pertechnetate per-rectal portal scintigraphy. J Nucl Med 1988;29(4):460–5.

63. Cole RC, Morandi F, Avenell J, et al. Trans-splenic portal scintigraphy in normal dogs. Vet Radiol Ultrasound 2005;46(2):146–52.

64. Landon BP, Abraham LA, Charles JA. Use of transcolonic portal scintigraphy to evaluate efficacy of cellophane banding of congenital extrahepatic portosystemic shunts in 16 dogs. Aust Vet J 2008;86(5):169–79.

65. Samii VF, Kyles AE, Long CD, et al. Evaluation of interoperator variance in shunt fraction calculation after transcolonic scintigraphy for diagnosis of portosystemic shunts in dogs and cats. J Am Vet Med Assoc 2001;218(7):1116–9.

66. Papazoglou LG, Monnet E, Seim HB III. Survival and prognostic indicators for dogs with intrahepatic portosystemic shunts: 32 cases (1990–2000). Vet Surg 2002;31(6):561–70.

67. Daniel GB, DeNovo RC, Sharp DS, et al. Portal streamlining as a cause of nonuniform hepatic distribution of sodium pertechnetate during per-rectal portal scintigraphy in the dog. Vet Radiol Ultrasound 2004;45(1):78–84.

68. Johnson CA, Armstrong PJ, Hauptman JG. Congenital portosystemic shunts in dogs: 46 cases (1979–1986). J Am Vet Med Assoc 1987;191(11):1478–83.

69. Morandi F, Sura PA, Sharp DS, et al. Scintigraphic features of multiple acquired portosystemic shunts using transplenic portal scintigraphy. Paper presented at: Annual Scientific Meeting of the American College of Veterinary Radiology; October 23, 2008, 2008; San Antonio, TX.

Index

Note: Page numbers of article titles are in **boldface** type.

A

Angiography, CT. See *Computed tomography (CT) angiography.*
Arterioportal fistulae, CT diagnosis of, 789–790
Artifact(s). See also specific types.
　digital radiographic, **689–709**. See also specific types and *Digital radiographic artifacts.*
　exposure, 695–700
　postexposure, 701–702
　preexposure, 689–694
　reading, 702–704
　workstation, 704–708
Atelectasis, on ultrasound of thorax, 743

B

Backscatter, 695
Border detection, 705

C

Calibration mask, 694
Cancer, on ultrasound of gastrointestinal tract, 757–758
Capture, digital, types of. See also *Digital capture.*
　comparison of, **677–688**
Cassette(s), upside-down, 695
Cassette-based digital radiography systems, 678–680
Cassette-less digital radiography systems, 680–682
Clipping, 706–707
Communication(s), digital imaging, in medicine, 674–675, 713–714
Computed tomography (CT)
　helical, in portosystemic shunt diagnosis, 784
　in hepatic vascular anomalies diagnosis, 787
　in portosystemic shunt diagnosis, **783–792**. See also *Portosystemic shunts, CT diagnosis of.*
　of arterioportal fistulae, 789–790
Computed tomography (CT) angiography
　in portosystemic shunt diagnosis, 784–785
　　technical aspects of, 785–786
　single- and dual-phase, of liver, 786
Crack(s), 690–691
Cranial mediastinum, ultrasound of, 736–738
CT. See *Computed tomography (CT).*

D

Dead pixels, 693–694
Debris, 702–703

Vet Clin Small Anim 39 (2009) 811–816
doi:10.1016/S0195-5616(09)00082-5
0195-5616/09/$ – see front matter © 2009 Elsevier Inc. All rights reserved.

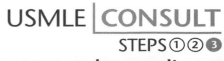

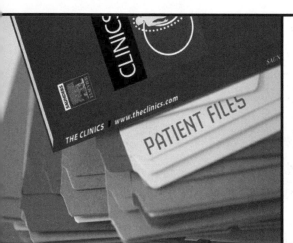
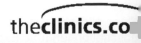

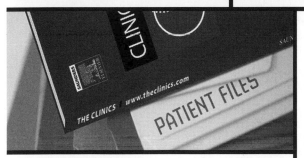

Moving?

Make sure your subscription moves with you!

To notify us of your new address, find your **Clinics Account Number** (located on your mailing label above your name), and contact customer service at:

E-mail: elspcs@elsevier.com

800-654-2452 (subscribers in the U.S. & Canada)
314-453-7041 (subscribers outside of the U.S. & Canada)

Fax number: 314-523-5170

Elsevier Periodicals Customer Service
11830 Westline Industrial Drive
St. Louis, MO 63146

*To ensure uninterrupted delivery of your subscription, please notify us at least 4 weeks in advance of move.